Two Sides of the Same Coin – Neurotransmitters in Health and Disease

Edited by Kaneez Fatima-Shad and Thomas Heinbockel

Published in London, United Kingdom

Two Sides of the Same Coin - Neurotransmitters in Health and Disease
http://dx.doi.org/10.5772/intechopen.1001719
Edited by Kaneez Fatima-Shad and Thomas Heinbockel

Contributors
Ammarah Baig, Andréia C.K. Fontana, Boris Aleksovski, Carmen Jimenez-Espinoza, Francisco Marcano Serrano, Javeria Tanveer, José González-Mora, Kaneez Fatima-Shad, Kanza Khan, Katelyn L. Reeb, Rhea Temmermand, Rukhsana Rubeen, Shazia Shakoor, Simran K. Gill, Vladimir Rendevski

First published in London, United Kingdom, 2025 by IntechOpen
IntechOpen is the global imprint of INTECHOPEN LIMITED, registered in England and Wales, registration number: 11086078, 167-169 Great Portland Street, London, W1W 5PF, United Kingdom

For EU product safety concerns: IN TECH d.o.o., Prolaz Marije Krucifikse Kozulić 3, 51000 Rijeka, Croatia, info@intechopen.com or visit our website at intechopen.com.

British Library Cataloguing-in-Publication Data
A catalogue record for this book is available from the British Library

Two Sides of the Same Coin - Neurotransmitters in Health and Disease
Edited by Kaneez Fatima-Shad and Thomas Heinbockel
p. cm.
Print ISBN 978-0-85466-656-0
Online ISBN 978-0-85466-655-3
eBook (PDF) ISBN 978-0-85466-657-7

Meet the editors

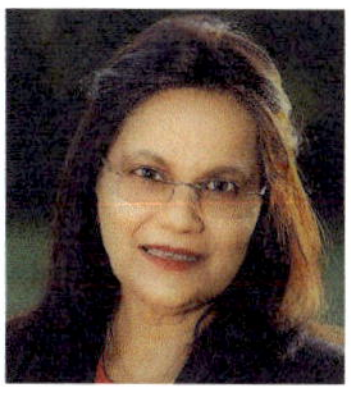

Dr. Kaneez Fatima Shad is an accomplished neuroscientist with over 35 years of teaching and research experience across Australia, the USA, UAE, Bahrain, Pakistan, and Brunei. She earned her Ph.D. from UNSW, completed a postdoc in the USA, and held senior academic roles at institutions worldwide. Currently based in Sydney, she is a Professor of Neuroscience and a visiting professor at UTS, UNSW, ACU, and Notre Dame. She has received over $3. 6 million in research funding and published extensively. Her work focuses on peripheral biomarkers for brain disorders, early stroke diagnosis, and supervision of thirty-five postgraduate students. Professor Shad is active in global neuroscience communities and serves as a regional representative and mentor for World Women in Neuroscience.

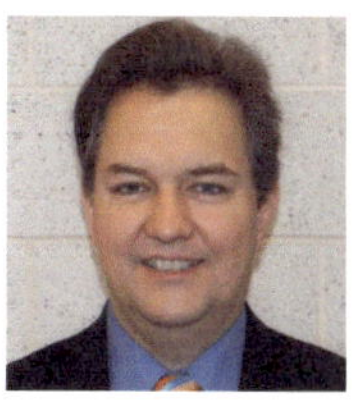

Thomas Heinbockel, Ph.D., is a professor in the Department of Anatomy, Howard University College of Medicine, Washington, DC. He holds an adjunct faculty position in both the Department of Anatomy and the Department of Physiology & Pharmacology at the University of Maryland School of Medicine, Baltimore, MD. His studies of the brain began during his master's thesis work at the Max Planck Institute for Behavioral Physiology in Seewiesen, Germany. Dr. Heinbockel earned a Ph.D. in Neuroscience at the University of Arizona, Tucson, AZ, USA. After graduating, he worked as a research associate at the Institute of Physiology, Otto von Guericke University, Magdeburg, Germany. Dr. Heinbockel's research focuses on understanding how the brain processes information in relation to neurological and psychiatric disorders. His laboratory at Howard University focuses on foundational and translational research topics, including drug development, the organization of the olfactory and limbic systems, neural signaling, and synaptic transmission in the central nervous system.

Contents

Preface

The human brain is often described as the most intricate structure in the known universe. At the heart of its complexity lie neurotransmitters—chemical messengers that shape thought, behavior, emotion, and cognition. Like two sides of the same coin, neurotransmitters play a dual role: they are essential for maintaining health and equilibrium, yet their imbalance or dysregulation can underlie a broad spectrum of neurological and psychiatric disorders.

This book, *Two Sides of the Same Coin – Neurotransmitters in Health and Disease*, seeks to explore the paradoxical nature of these powerful molecules. It presents a comprehensive yet accessible journey through the physiological roles of neurotransmitters in normal brain function, while also delving into how their alterations contribute to diseases such as depression, schizophrenia, Alzheimer's disease, stroke, and other neurodegenerative and neurovascular conditions.

Drawing upon decades of research and clinical insight, this volume bridges the gap between fundamental neuroscience and translational medicine. It is intended for students, researchers, and clinicians who wish to deepen their understanding of the chemical language of the brain—both in harmony and in disruption.

The title reflects the central thesis of this book: that neurotransmitters are neither inherently beneficial nor harmful, but context-dependent agents of change. Their duality is what makes them both fascinating and vital to understanding the human condition.

We are grateful to IntechOpen for initiating this book project and for asking us to serve as its editors. Many thanks are due to Ms. Valentina Jolic at IntechOpen for guiding us through the publication process and for advancing the book in a timely manner. Thanks are due to all contributors of this book for taking the time to first write a chapter proposal, compose their chapter, and, lastly, make the requested revisions to it.

Dr. Heinbockel would like to thank his wife, Dr. Vonnie D.C. Shields, Professor at Towson University, Towson, MD, and their son, Torben Heinbockel, for the time he was able to spend working on this book project during the past year. He is grateful to his parents, Erich and Renate Heinbockel, for their continuous support and interest in his work over many years.

Hopefully, all contributors will continue their research, facing many intellectual challenges and exploring exciting new directions. We hope that this work not only informs but also inspires further inquiry into the delicate balance that governs brain chemistry, and ultimately, human life.

Dr. Kaneez Fatima-Shad
Professor,
University of Technology Sydney,
Sydney, Australia

Thomas Heinbockel, Ph.D.
Department of Anatomy,
Howard University College of Medicine,
Washington, DC, USA

Chapter 1

Introductory Chapter: Glutamate, a Double Edge Sword

Kaneez Fatima-Shad

1. Introduction

Glutamate is a major excitatory neurotransmitter responsible for synaptic plasticity and other essential processes, such as learning and memory, in the central nervous system [1]. This amazing amino acid seems to be involved in the biosynthesis of almost all proteins and nucleic acids [2]. Glutamate regulates various metabolic pathways and signaling mechanisms by interacting with both its ionic and metabotropic receptors [3].

2. Dual nature of glutamate

Glutamate is a molecule that can have both positive and negative effects on the body, so it can be considered both "*wonderful*" and "*dreadful*" in certain situations.

2.1 Wonderful molecule

Nonessential amino acid glutamate cannot cross the blood-brain barrier and is synthesized in the presynaptic neuron from glutamine *via* the mitochondrial enzyme glutaminase. Non-neuronal cells, such as astrocytes, also produce glutamate *via* the enzyme pyruvate carboxylase. This synthesis increases during brain activation, for example, during memory formation [4].

2.1.1 Neuromodulator

Huang et al. [5] demonstrated that type III gustatory cells are stimulated by low concentrations of glutamate and release serotonin, which in turn reduces ATP release from type II gustatory cells. ATP is known to be an afferent transmitter in taste buds.

2.1.2 Metabolic regulator

In many organisms, the amino acid glutamate is not only involved in the synthesis of proteins, nucleotides, and other amino acids but also plays a role in nitrogen assimilation and catabolism of certain amines. For these reasons, it is often referred to as "metabolic hub" [6]. In numerous metabolic pathways, including the tricarboxylic acid (TCA) cycle and the glutamine-glutamate cycle glutamate acts as an important metabolic intermediate. It synthesizes the inhibitory neurotransmitter gamma-aminobutyric acid (GABA) along with other important molecules.

2.2 Dreadful molecule

Glutamate is involved in the onset of many cardiovascular, cerebrovascular, neurodegenerative, and psychiatric disorders such as hypertension, stroke, Alzheimer's disease, and schizophrenia.

2.2.1 Hypertension

Expression of different subunits in pre and postsynaptic NMDA receptors dysregulate blood pressure. Interaction between the neuropeptide orexin and glutamatergic receptor N-Methyl-D Aspartate (NMDA) was recently observed [7]. They also identified that the resultant molecules produced from the increased influx of calcium ions through NMDA receptors (NMDARs) could serve as predictive biomarkers of hypertension.

2.2.2 Stroke and Alzheimer's disease

Qin et al. [8], demonstrated that increased activities of excitatory amino acid, along with glucose deprivation and ischemic conditions, cause excitotoxicity and neuronal death. The sequence of events in such conditions includes an excess of calcium, leading to ionic imbalance, membrane depolarization, and unrestricted activation of glutamatergic receptors, mitochondrial dysfunction, and alterations in gene expression [9].

This glutamate-gated excitotoxicity is recognized as a major contributing factor to the early stages of Alzheimer's disease and ischemic stroke [10].

2.2.3 Schizophrenia

We and others observed that human platelets mimic neuronal receptors, such as NMDA and serotonin type 3 receptors, as well as ionic currents. Experiments performed on platelets from both healthy individuals and patients with schizophrenia revealed a very similar baseline electrophysiological profile.

Significant differences in the ionic currents were observed when serotonin was applied to the platelets from normal individuals and patients with schizophrenia. We found that the serotonin-induced currents in platelets from patients with schizophrenia were four times greater than those in normal individuals, indicating a marked difference in the sensitivity and distribution of the serotonin receptors between the two groups.

We also observed that D-serine at micromolar concentrations decreased the amplitude and sensitivity of serotonin receptors present in the platelets of patients with schizophrenia and that D-serine can reduce 5-HT3 receptor sensitivity, bringing the values closer to those of normal subjects [11].

3. Conclusion

The balance between the production and consumption of glutamate is essential for retaining homeostasis of excitatory neurotransmission in both the brain and the body.

DOI: http://dx.doi.org/10.5772/intechopen.1006727

Author details

Kaneez Fatima-Shad
University of Technology, Sydney, Australia

*Address all correspondence to: ftmshad@gmail.com

References

[1] Pal MM. Glutamate: The master neurotransmitter and its implications in chronic stress and mood disorders. Frontiers in Human Neuroscience. 2021;**15**:1-4. DOI: 10.3389/fnhum.2021.722323

[2] Wakabayashi Y, Yamada E, Hasegawa T, Yamada R. Enzymological evidence for the indispensability of small intestine in the synthesis of arginine from glutamate. I. Pyrroline-5-carboxylate synthase. Archives of Biochemistry and Biophysics. 1991;**291**:1-8

[3] Szczurowska E, Mares P. NMDA and AMPA receptors: Development and status epilepticus. Physiological Research. 2013;**62**(Suppl. 1):S21-S38

[4] Bonvento G, Bolaños JP. Astrocyte-neuron metabolic cooperation shapes brain activity. Cell Metabolism. 2021;**33**(8):1546-1564. DOI: 10.1016/j.cmet.2021.07.006

[5] Huang YJ, Maruyama Y, Dvoryanchikov G, Pereira E, Chaudhari N, Roper SD. The role of pannexin 1 hemichannels in ATP release and cell-cell communication in mouse taste buds. Proceedings of the National Academy of Sciences of the United States of America. 2007;**104**:6436-6441

[6] Walker MC, van der Donk WA. The many roles of glutamate in metabolism. Journal of Industrial Microbiology & Biotechnology. 2016;**43**(2-3):419-430. DOI: 10.1007/s10295-015-1665-y

[7] Shad K, F, Abdi F, Simpson AM. Early predictive biomarkers for hypertension using human Fetal astrocytes. Journal of Vascular Medicine & Surgeries. 2024:1-8. DOI: 10.47363/JVMS/2024(2)109

[8] Qin C, Yang S, Chu YH, Zhang H, Pang XW, Chen L, et al. Signaling pathways involved in ischemic stroke: Molecular mechanisms and therapeutic interventions. Signal Transduction and Targeted Therapy. 2022;**7**:215

[9] Kirdajova DB, Kriska J, Tureckova J, Anderova M. Ischemia-triggered glutamate excitotoxicity from the perspective of glial cells. Frontiers in Cellular Neuroscience. 2020;**19**:51

[10] Tushar KD, Ganesh BP, Fatima-Shad K. Common Signaling pathways involved in Alzheimer’s disease and stroke: Two faces of the same coin. Journal of Alzheimer's Disease Reports. 2023;7(1):381-398. DOI: 10.3233/ADR-220108

[11] Fatima-Shad K. Effect of D-serine on the serotonin receptors of human platelets. Experimental Brain Research. 2006;**173**:353-356. DOI: 10.1007/s00221-006-0496-5

Chapter 2

Glutamate Signaling and NMDA Receptor Dynamics in Healthy Aging and Alzheimer's Disease

Ammarah Baig, Javeria Tanveer, Rukhsana Rubeen, Shazia Shakoor, Kanza Khan and Kaneez Fatima-Shad

Abstract

This chapter provides a comprehensive overview of glutamate, the primary excitatory neurotransmitter in the central nervous system, and its interaction with N-methyl-D-aspartate receptors (NMDARs), pivotal for synaptic plasticity, neural transmission, and cognitive functions. We highlight the critical role of glutamate signaling in aging and Alzheimer's disease (AD), emphasizing how dysregulated glutamatergic activity contributes to neuronal damage and neurodegeneration through excitotoxicity. A central focus is the pathological overactivation of extrasynaptic NMDARs, which elevates intracellular calcium levels and triggers neurotoxic cascades involving oxidative stress, mitochondrial dysfunction, and apoptosis. Furthermore, hallmark AD pathologies, such as Tau tangles and amyloid-beta (Aβ) plaques, exacerbate glutamate dysregulation, enhancing NMDAR-mediated calcium influx and excitotoxicity. The chapter also explores the role of glutamate transporters in cognitive decline, highlighting age-related impairments in the glutamate-glutamine cycle that reduce extracellular glutamate clearance. Therapeutic strategies targeting glutamate homeostasis and NMDAR signaling may offer novel avenues for mitigating synaptic dysfunction and improving outcomes in AD and age-related cognitive decline. This review aims to lay the foundation for developing targeted interventions to address these neurodegenerative processes.

Keywords: neurodegenerative diseases, Alzheimer's disease, glutamate receptors, cognitive decline, NMDA receptor

1. Introduction

Glutamate is the most abundant free amino acid and the primary excitatory neurotransmitter in the mammalian brain, situated at the intersection of multiple metabolic pathways. It plays a crucial role in fundamental brain processes, including synaptic plasticity, which underlies learning, memory formation, and the development of neural networks. Additionally, glutamate is essential for regulating motor control through its involvement in neuronal circuits within the basal ganglia [1].

However, under pathological conditions, dysregulated glutamate signaling can induce excitotoxicity, contributing to neuronal damage and is implicated in various neurological disorders, including Alzheimer's disease (AD).

1.1 Glutamate synthesis, release, and metabolism

Glutamate is classified as a non-essential amino acid because it is synthesized endogenously within the central nervous system (CNS) through the glutamate-glutamine cycle. Although glutamate has limited direct access from the bloodstream to the brain, neighboring glial cells release glutamine, which is taken up by neuronal presynaptic terminals via excitatory amino acid transporters (EAATs). Within the presynaptic terminals, glutamine is converted to glutamate by the mitochondrial enzyme glutaminase. The synthesized glutamate is then packaged into synaptic vesicles through the action of vesicular glutamate transporters (VGLUTs). Upon the arrival of an action potential, voltage-gated ion channels in the presynaptic membrane open, allowing Na^+ and Ca^{2+} influx, which triggers the release of glutamate into the synaptic cleft. The released glutamate interacts with receptors on the postsynaptic neuron to mediate excitatory neurotransmission, playing a critical role in synaptic communication and neuronal signaling [2]. The influx of Ca^{2+} triggers the fusion of glutamate-containing vesicles with the presynaptic membrane, leading to the release of glutamate into the synaptic cleft. To prevent excitotoxicity and maintain synaptic homeostasis, excitatory amino acid transporters (EAATs) rapidly clear glutamate from the synaptic cleft, transporting it into either glial cells or presynaptic terminals. In glial cells, glutamate is enzymatically converted back into glutamine-by-glutamine synthetase. This glutamine is subsequently shuttled back to neurons, where it is reconverted to glutamate, completing the glutamate-glutamine cycle. The coordinated interaction between neurons and glial cells ensures a continuous and efficient supply of glutamate for neurotransmission while preventing excessive extracellular accumulation [3]. See **Figure 1**.

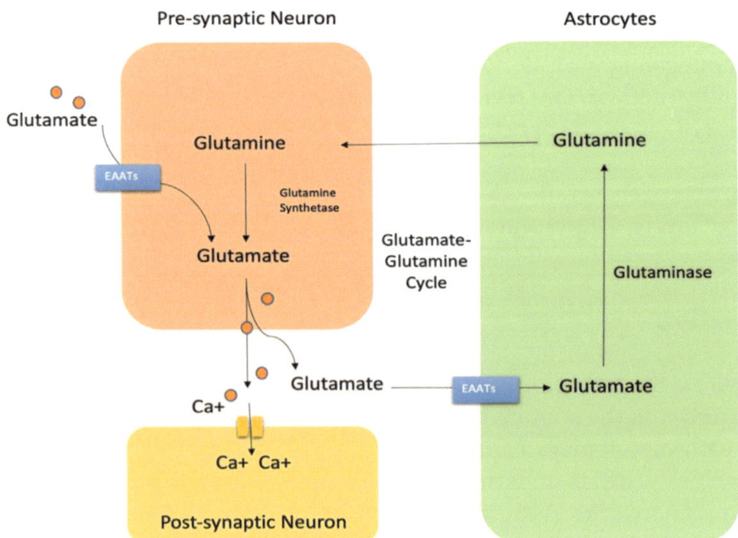

Figure 1.
Simple representation of glutamate-glutamine cycle.

1.2 Glutamate receptors

Alpha-amino-3-hydroxy-5-methyl-4-isoxazole propionic acid (AMPA), N-methyl-D-aspartate (NMDA), and kainate receptors are the three main types of ionotropic glutamate receptors responsible for fast excitatory neurotransmission in the central nervous system (CNS). While they share a similar structural framework, they differ in amino acid composition, subunit assembly, and agonist sensitivity. These receptors are distributed across pre-synaptic, post-synaptic, and extra-synaptic regions, contributing to synaptic transmission and plasticity.

AMPA receptors primarily mediate rapid synaptic responses, while NMDA receptors are involved in slower, calcium-dependent synaptic responses essential for synaptic plasticity. Kainate receptors, formed from distinct genes (GluR5-7, KA-1, and KA-2), are widely distributed throughout the brain and have been implicated in processes such as epileptogenesis and cell death, although their precise physiological roles remain less well understood [4].

In addition to ionotropic receptors, there are eight metabotropic glutamate receptors (mGluR1–8) belonging to the G-protein-coupled receptor family, which modulate neuronal excitability and synaptic transmission over slower timescales. Metabotropic receptors, on the other hand, lack ion channels. Glutamate binds to a metabotropic receptor and activates an intracellular G-protein, which starts signaling cascades that indirectly affect postsynaptic ion channels. In contrast to ionotropic receptors, these receptors have a slower postsynaptic response and can either increase or decrease excitability [5].

Group I mGluRs are located on postsynaptic membranes and are thought to improve responses mediated by ionotropic receptors. On the other hand, group II and III mGluRs, which are mainly found on presynaptic membranes, might act as auto receptors and control glutamate release by means of feedback processes.

This comprehensive distribution and functional diversity highlight the central role of glutamate receptors in both normal CNS function and pathological conditions. (Refer to **Figure 2** and **Table 1**).

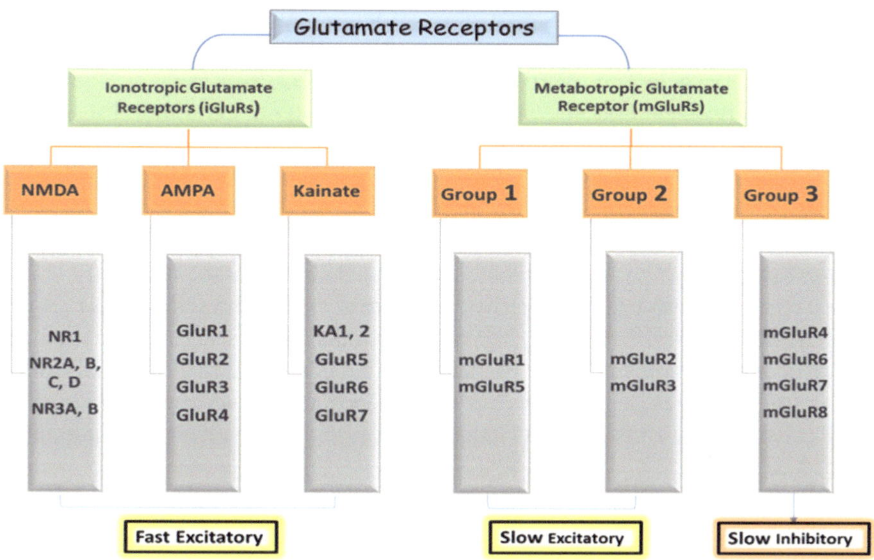

Figure 2.
Classification of glutamate receptors.

Receptor type	Subtypes	Key features	Signaling mechanism
iGluRs	NMDA, AMPA, KA	Fast synaptic transmission, ion flow	Ligand-gated ion channels
mGluRs	mGluR1—mGluR8	Modulation, plasticity, slow effects	G protein-coupled signaling

Table 1.
A comparison table of iGluR/mGluR properties.

1.3 Changes in glutamate levels during aging

With aging, the brain function declines [6], which is associated by a decrease in mitochondrial energy production in the thalamus-cortical neurons, reflected by a reduced rate of the glutamate-glutamine cycle [7]. During physiological aging memory function also tends to decline, due to hypo glutamatergic activities.

In rodents [8, 9] and in humans, not necessarily in all humans, there is a decline of cerebral glutamate levels with the age was observed via proton MR spectroscopy (1H-MRS) especially in the cortical areas [6, 7, 10–12]. Studies were made to quantify glutamine within the cortical region showed subtle results in healthy aging [6, 10].

1.4 Glutamate and neurodegeneration

Glutamate has gained significant interest from neurologists because of its potential role in acute and chronic neurodegenerative disorders. The following three basic underlying mechanisms were suggested:

1. Exogenous dietary glutamate (for instance, MSG compounds) can cause excitotoxicity by stimulating glutamate receptors.

2. In conditions such as cerebral ischemia and brain injury, glutamate released endogenously from neurons contributes to acute neurodegeneration.

3. Excitotoxicity i.e. hyperactivity of glutamatergic receptors can contribute to cell death in neurodegenerative disorders like ALS (Amyotrophic lateral sclerosis), Huntington's disease, Parkinson's disease and Alzheimer's disease [13].

1.5 Glutamate dysfunction in Alzheimer's disease (AD)

The leading cause of pathogenesis of Alzheimer's disease is excitotoxicity of glutamate receptors, especially N-methyl-D-aspartate receptors (NMDARs) [14]. The underlying mechanism of this excitotoxicity is disruption of astrocyte mediated glutamate uptake and excessive release of glutamate in presynaptic terminals induced by beta amyloid plaques [15]. Studies have revealed that the overexcitation, leads to influx of calcium ions, causing neuronal loss and cognitive decline of Alzheimer's disease [16, 17].

This chapter offers a comprehensive review of glutamate, the central nervous system's primary excitatory neurotransmitter and its complex interaction with N-methyl-D-aspartate receptors (NMDARs), critical to synaptic plasticity, neural transmission, and cognitive health. The chapter starts with a description of normal physiological glutamatergic signaling and its significance to healthy brain health, followed by discussion of how this system gets dysregulated with age and in Alzheimer's disease (AD). A centralized focus is given to the pathological overactivation of extrasynaptic NMDARs, which triggers a cascade of intracellular calcium overloading, oxidative stress, mitochondrial damage, and apoptosis which are major drivers of neuronal loss and cognitive decline. The chapter also borrows from nascent knowledge of how common AD pathologies, i.e., amyloid-beta (Aβ) deposition and tau pathology, lead to glutamate-mediated excitotoxicity. Furthermore, we assess the loss of glutamate transporter function and the impaired glutamate-glutamine cycle, especially in the aging brain, that further aggravate extracellular glutamate accumulation. On this mechanistic foundation, the chapter discusses current and experimental treatment strategies to restore glutamate homeostasis, modulate NMDAR function, and maintain synaptic health. By integrating these lines of evidence, this chapter seeks not only to explain the multifaceted role of glutamatergic dysfunction in AD but also to lay bare its therapeutic potential, paving the way for future intervention into this critical neurotransmitter system.

2. Glutamate transporters dysfunction in Alzheimer's disease

The concentrations of extracellular glutamate are also regulated by glutamate transporters, expressed on neurons and astrocytes. The glutamate transporters play a critical role in preserving synaptic homeostasis, by withdrawing the excess amount of glutamate from the cleft of the synaptic membrane. Glutamate transporter failure is a major cause of excitotoxicity and neuronal injury in neurodegenerative diseases like Alzheimer's [13].

There are two types of glutamate transporters involved in the removal of extra levels of glutamate from synaptic cleft [18]. These EAAT1 and EAAT2T are integral membrane proteins, responsible for clearing excess glutamate from the synaptic cleft into glial cells and neurons [19]. EAAT1 is mostly found in cerebellum and EAAT2 is present on astrocytes in the cerebral cortex and hippocampus to maintain the glutamate level by transporting the excess amount of glutamate in the brain [20].

In AD, the dysregulation of glutamate transporters, specifically EAAT2, results in high extracellular glutamate levels due to decreased astrocytic glutamate uptake and resultant excitotoxicity [21]. Genetic variations of EAAT2 is associated with lower glutamate uptake, contributing to the onset of Alzheimer's disease [22].

2.1 Consequences of impaired glutamate clearance in Alzheimer's disease

The inadequate activities of glutamate transporters i.e. Excitatory Amino Acid Transporters (EAATs) may lead to symptoms of Alzheimer's disease. EAAT1 and EAAT2 transporters maintaining the homeostasis of glutamate levels in the brain [23, 24].

EAAT1 and EAAT2 are predominantly localized on astrocytes, with EAAT1 highly expressed in the cerebellum and EAAT2 in the hippocampus. Their activity prevents excessive glutamate accumulation, thereby avoiding excitotoxicity [25, 26], EAAT2 is not exclusively astrocytic; it has also been detected in neurons, particularly in the hippocampus and retina [27]. Upon glutamate release from presynaptic neurons, a substantial portion diffuses out of the synaptic cleft. Astrocytic EAATs, especially EAAT2, are critical in clearing this excess glutamate, preventing spillover to neighboring synapses and avoiding overactivation of extrasynaptic NMDA receptors. This regulatory mechanism is disrupted in AD.

Amyloid β, a hallmark of AD, has been shown to reduce both EAAT1 and EAAT2 function and expression in rat hippocampal and cortical astrocytes. Human studies have similarly documented decreased expression of these transporters in the hippocampi and cortices of AD patients, correlating with reduced glutamate uptake [27]. While the role of EAAT2 has been relatively well characterized, EAAT1's involvement remains ambiguous. Some studies suggest increased EAAT1 expression in the hippocampus of AD patients, potentially as a compensatory response [26], while others note reduced expression in platelets, indicating systemic glutamate dysregulation [28].

EAAT2 alterations are more consistent: protein levels and function are significantly decreased in the AD frontal cortex despite stable mRNA levels, suggesting post-transcriptional regulation problems [29]. This downregulation is linked with astrocyte dysfunction, increased gliosis, and is associated with, but not fully explained by, amyloid and tau burden [29, 30]. Notably, both astrocytic and neuronal EAAT2 are implicated in memory, with astrocytic deficiency being more strongly tied to AD pathology [31]. Peripheral changes have also been observed, such as reductions in platelet EAAT1 and EAAT3 during aging and AD, indicating potential peripheral biomarkers [28].

Mechanistically, multiple factors link EAAT dysfunction to AD. Neuroinflammation, driven by microglial and astrocyte activation, alters EAAT1/2 expression and impairs synaptic plasticity [32]. Moreover, beta-amyloid disrupts insulin/Akt/EAAT signaling pathways, lowering EAAT protein levels and potentially promoting excitotoxic damage—a process reversible with insulin treatment [33]. Altered EAAT2 is also associated with abnormal expression of the amyloid precursor protein (APP), linking transporter dysfunction with amyloidogenesis [29].

Given that EAAT expression is influenced by neuronal and endothelial signaling, the decline in transporter function in AD may stem from disrupted intercellular communication. Thus, targeting EAAT1 and EAAT2 for therapeutic upregulation holds promise for mitigating glutamate toxicity and slowing disease progression.

In addition, the release of excitotoxicity leads to the generation of reactive microglial cells, which produce cytokines resulting in neuroinflammation [34] and the generation of the neurofibrillary tangles. (Refer to **Table 2** for a brief summary of the role of EAAT1/2 in AD pathology.

2.1.1 Amyloid-beta (Aβ) toxicity

The neuronal death and synaptic dysfunction in Alzheimer's disease is mainly due to abnormal accumulation of amyloid-beta (Aβ) peptides, which are produced by the proteolytic cleavage of amyloid precursor protein (APP) [35]. The primary pathogenic

Protein	Gene	Localization	Alterations in AD
EAAT1	*SLC1A3*	Astrocytes (including Bergmann & Müller glia) Predominant in cerebellum Present in retina [27].	Upregulated in the medial temporal lobe (suggesting compensation) [26] Downregulated in platelets and some brain areas [28].
EAAT2	*SLC1A2*	Astrocytes (and some sparse neurons) Predominant in hippocampus and cortex [27].	Reduced protein levels and function in AD brains [29] Post-transcriptional regulation issues despite stable mRNA levels. Associated with gliosis and abnormal amyloid precursor protein APP dysregulation [30, 31].

Table 2.
Localization and alterations of EAAT 1/2 in AD pathology.

characteristic of AD, insoluble plaques, can be formed by the oligomerization and aggregation of these peptides leading to severe neurotoxicity and synaptic function, especially in soluble forms [36]. They cause synaptic depression and disrupt long-term potentiation (LTP), a neuronal process that underlies learning and memory [37]. Furthermore, Aβ oligomers exacerbate excitotoxicity by interfering with the release of neurotransmitters, especially glutamate [38]. In addition to causing oxidative stress, mitochondrial malfunction, and disruption of intracellular signaling cascades, Aβ toxicity also results in neuronal damage and cell death [39]. Researchers have also suggested that Aβ peptides can stimulate astrocytes and microglia, resulting in neuroinflammatory reactions that worsens neurodegeneration [39]. Postmortem examinations of brains affected by Alzheimer's disease have consistently revealed indications of underlying neuroinflammation. These alterations are indicative of the presence of activated microglia surrounding amyloid plaques and elevated levels of pro-inflammatory cytokines [40]. It is vital to address the underlying processes of Aβ toxicity to explore effective treatment options, which should be aimed at reducing its deleterious effects and stopping the course of Alzheimer's disease.

2.1.2 Tau pathology

Alzheimer's disease cognitive impairment and disease progression are significantly correlated with tau pathology [41]. It is suggested that the underlying mechanism causing neurodegeneration of Alzheimer's disease is abnormal accumulation of hyperphosphorylated Tau proteins.

Tau protein is present in neuronal axons, where it is responsible for intracellular facilitation and stabilization of microtubules. In Alzheimer's disease, the tau proteins become phosphorylated leading to accumulation of neurofibrillary tangles (NFTs) which cause disruption of regular cellular activities like synaptic dysfunction, interference with axonal transport, neuronal damage and cell death [42, 43]. Transgenic animal models have been used in studies to show that overexpression of mutant tau protein recapitulates important characteristics of the pathogenesis of Alzheimer's disease, such as neurodegeneration and synaptic dysfunction [44, 45].

3. The NMDAR paradox

In the central nervous system (CNS), a multitude of excitatory neurotransmission is regulated, via the vesicular discharge of glutamates stimulating ionotropic glutamate receptors (iGluRs) and pre- and postsynaptic G-protein-coupled metabotropic glutamate receptors [46].

N-methyl-d-aspartate receptor (NMDAR) is distinguished from other glutamate receptors, for an increased Ca^{2+} permeability extracellular Mg^{2+} blockade in a voltage dependent manner, as well as the necessity of two co agonists binding to the agonist recognition site i.e. glutamate and glycine (or d-serine), to activate the channel [47].

3.1 Localization of NMDAR

In growing brain circuits, NMDARs placed post synaptically serve as detector, while NMDARs located presynaptic-ally mediate synaptic transmission and activity-dependent synaptic plasticity [48].

The temporal cortex and hippocampus of developing brains exhibit modest expression of the NR1, NR2A, and NR2C subunits of the NMDA receptor, but in neonates, this expression is distributed across the brain. Although NR2B is hardly noticeable in adults, the NR2B subunit is minimally expressed in the fetal hippocampal and temporal cortex [49]. From weeks 7–21, NR3A levels plummet and rapidly increases post-birth, and decline gradually into adulthood [50], and NR3B levels rise as postnatal development advances, in adulthood, NR3A remains low while NR3B stays high. NR1 expression is low during gestation and escalates until adolescence [51]. Long-term potentiation (LTP) and long-term depression (LTD), two processes underpinning synaptic plasticity, depend on NMDA receptors, which are the principal mediators of calcium signaling in hippocampal neurons [52]. Both NR2A along with NR2B subunits are paramount for inducing of LTD and LTP [53]. See **Figure 3**.

3.2 Synaptic and extra synaptic NMDAR

Extra synaptic NMDARs are the ones that are found outside of the synapse, on the sides of spines or dendrites. They also cluster at sites of contact with nearby structures i.e. axons, axon terminals, or glia [54], while synaptic NMDARs are situated on the postsynaptic membrane of the synapse. When glutamate binds to NMDARs, it causes an unfolding chain of events resulting in the opening of the receptor's ion channel, letting calcium ions (Ca^{2+}) pass through the postsynaptic neurons. In conclusion, Ca^{2+} excess is not the only factor determining neurotoxicity; rather, Ca^{2+} influx through NMDARs positioned beyond the synapse is particularly detrimental to neurons [49]. See **Figure 4**.

Aβ, a protein linked to Alzheimer's disease, initiates extra synaptic NMDA receptors (NMDARs) in neurons, causing astrocytes to release glutamate. The activation of these extra synaptic NMDARs could bring about a drop in miniature excitatory postsynaptic currents (mEPSCs), which are small, spontaneous shifts in the electrical characteristics of neurons at synapses. A drop in mEPSCs may indicate early synaptic damage, contributing to the course of Alzheimer's disease [55].

Synaptic NMDARs are impeded by d-serine degradation, the magnitude of LTP expression is reduced, whereas glycine degradation has no effect on LTP, implying that synaptic NMDARs play an important role in LTP but not extra synaptic. Conversely, both synaptic and extra synaptic NMDARs are necessary for LTD [56].

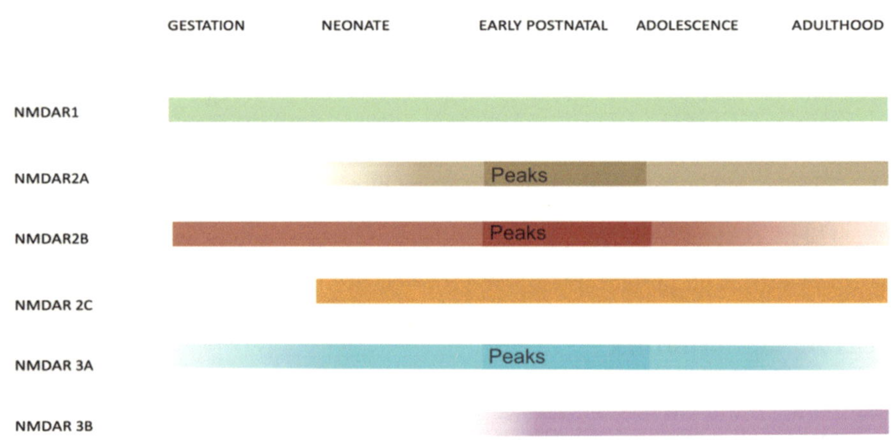

Figure 3.
Developmental timeline of NMDAR receptor subunits.

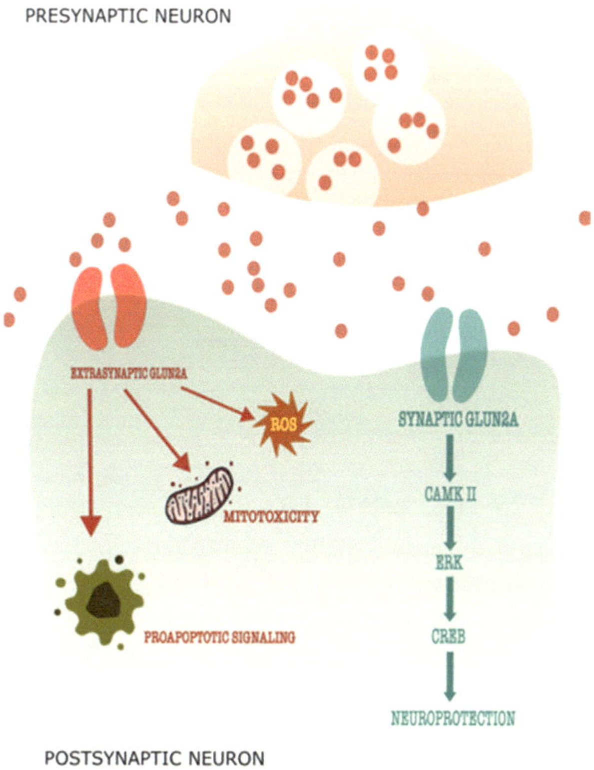

Figure 4.
Postsynaptic changes brought about in a cell by synaptic and extra synaptic receptors.

3.3 Activation of NMDAR

During the resting state, there is a voltage-dependent blockade on NMDA pore by extracellular Mg^{2+}, the block (**Figure 5**) is released upon depolarization of the receptor, hence, the activation is dependent on the membrane potential at the post synaptic end and the frequency of Glutamate being released from the presynaptic terminal, rendering these receptors with a unique potential to simultaneously respond to both presynaptic glutamate release and postsynaptic depolarization with a slow synaptic current, resulting in the ample influx of external Ca^{2+} into the dendritic spine [57, 58]. Consequently, increasing intracellular Ca^{2+} signals the initiation of the cascade of events leading to a multitude of changes in the postsynaptic neuron, resulting in short-term or long-term changes in synaptic strength and excitatory glutamatergic neurotransmission which is critical for survival of neurons and synaptic plasticity [46, 52, 59–62]. The duration and frequency of the activation of synaptic NMDA receptor influences the nature of these changes [63, 64]. Although apparently the synapsis of the NMDAR seems to be directly affected by the glutamate, but the activation through glutamate is only temporary, owing to the continuous presence of extracellular glycine (or d-serine) at a fairly constant concentration [65–67].

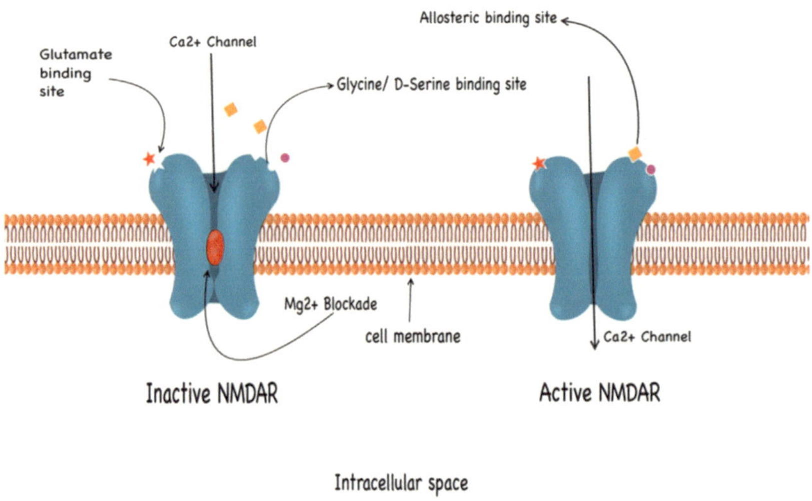

Figure 5.
A comparison of NMDAR in both active and inactive state.

3.4 The tripartite glutamate synapse

The presynaptic terminal, postsynaptic spine, and astrocytic cell engage during glutamate-mediated synaptic transmission. Glutamate is stored in synaptic vesicles by presynaptic glutamate transporters (VGLUTs) [68]. The calcium channels open, allowing calcium to enter, which discharges glutamate into the synapse upon the fusion of the vesicles with the membrane. Once the presynaptic neuron depolarizes glutamate thereafter activates receptors on postsynaptic and presynaptic neurons, as well as on the astrocytes, increasing internal calcium levels in astrocytes results in the release of neurotransmitters that dictate synaptic strength [69].

Glutamate is extracted from the extracellular environment into the astrocytes by excitatory amino acid transporters 1/2 (EAAT1/2) in astrocytes and EAAT2/5 in the presynaptic terminal and stored in vesicles where glutamine synthase turns glutamate into glutamine. The glutamine is transported back to glutamatergic neurons and converted back into glutamate [70]. This glutamate and a co-agonist which can either be glycine or D-serine, binds to the postsynaptic neuron, thereby, depolarizing it, opens the NMDA channels, letting Ca^{2+} influx through the postsynaptic terminal. This can trigger signals which support long-term potentiation (LTP), a process essential for learning and memory [71]. However, the surplus of Ca^{2+} through prolonged stimulation of NMDAR is deleterious to the cell [72].

Glutamate transport systems could shut off excitatory signaling, transport glutamate to extra synaptic receptors, and protect neurons from excitotoxic damage. The sodium-dependent EAATs mediate most of the glutamate transport in the CNS, notably during excitatory transmission. When glutamate release surpasses the capacity of astrocyte clearance systems, or EAAT expression drops, excitotoxicity may occur. Both chronic and acute neurological disorders have been linked to GLT-1/EAAT-2 dysfunction or reduced expression (**Figure 6**) [73].

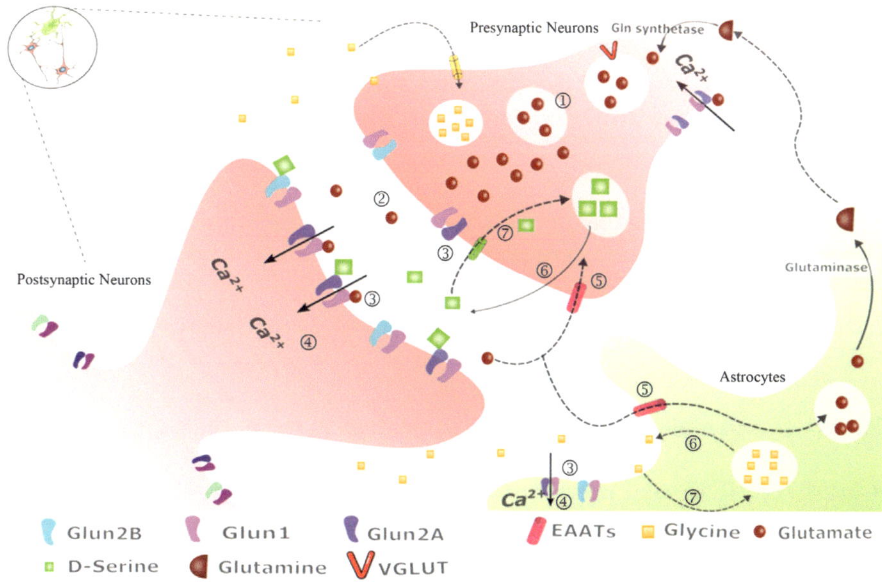

Figure 6.
Overview of the tripartite glutamate synapse. (1) Glutamate is stored in presynaptic vesicles and released into the synaptic cleft. (2) It binds to postsynaptic NMDARs, triggering calcium influx and action potential propagation. (3) Glutamate uptake occurs via EAAT transporters in astrocytes and presynaptic terminals. (4) Glycine and D-serine, released by neurons and astrocytes, modulate receptor activation and are recycled through transporters.

3.4.1 Role of NMDAR in Alzheimer's disease

Alzheimer's disease (AD) is the most common neurodegenerative disorder, contributing to cognitive decline and memory loss in almost 40 million people worldwide [74]. AD primarily affects the hippocampus and neocortex—critical regions for cognitive function and memory.

Features of AD

- Synaptic loss
- Deposition of Aβ plaques
- Neurofibrillary tangles (NFTs)
- Hyperphosphorylated tau.

These pathological features contribute to oxidative stress and NMDAR activation, leading to glutamatergic dysfunction and Ca^{2+} dyshomeostasis, both of which play significant roles in AD, particularly in its early stages. Recent studies highlight the involvement of tripartite glutamatergic synapses in AD pathogenesis [75]. The resulting high Ca^{2+} influx and free radical generation further phosphorylate tau, leading to mitochondrial dysfunction, permeability transition pore activation, cytochrome c release, ATP depletion, and ROS formation [49]. Multiple regulatory sites within the tripartite synapse modulate extracellular glutamate levels and are sensitive to

AD-related changes. Interruptions in these synapses contribute to AD pathogenesis through:

1. Overstimulation of NMDARs, contributing to excessive intracellular Ca^{2+} and subsequent cell death [76].

2. Low during gestation Impaired astrocytic glutamate clearance or reduced expression of EAATs, leading to excitotoxicity [73].

3. Dysfunction or downregulation of GLT-1/EAAT-2, which may exacerbate AD [73].

3.5 Pathways and molecular mechanisms involved in the pathology of AD

3.5.1 CREB (cAMP response element binding protein) and synaptic plasticity

CREB is the prototypical signal-regulated transcription factor essential for long-term potentiation (LTP), Within the hippocampus, CREB-mediated gene expression associated with synaptic plasticity, learning and memory, Phosphorylation of CREB at residue ser-133 is particularly important for its transcriptional activity, which is decreased in AD [74].

3.5.2 Activation of CREB

A broad range of signaling processes can trigger the phosphorylation of CREB, which leads to its activation. Some of these processes include an increase in intracellular Ca^{2+} through NMDARs, by growth factors activating receptor tyrosine kinase. This calcium entry through synaptic NMDARs induces CREB phosphorylation and Brain-derived neurotrophic factor (BDNF) expression, while extra synaptic NMDARs shuts-off the CREB pathway [77].

3.5.3 Amyloid-β (Aβ) and CREB

Amyloid-β (Aβ) accumulation in Alzheimer's disease is linked to memory loss, synaptic dysfunction, and a decrease in brain-derived neurotrophic factor (BDNF). Aβ dephosphorylates CREB through inactivation of protein kinase A (PKA) and thus inhibits of long-term potentiation (LTP) generation [78].

3.5.4 Jacob and synaptic plasticity

Jacob is a caldendrin-binding protein in the brain that is localized to the nucleus, it promotes synaptic contact loss while impeding CREB phosphorylation. Elevated NMDAR activity has been shown to aid in Jacob's nuclear accumulation [43]. Cell death or cell survival and synaptic plasticity depend on the level of Jacob phosphorylation. Upon synaptic NMDAR stimulation, phosphorylated Jacob is carried to the nucleus and is believed to be associated with neuroprotection while non-phosphorylated Jacob, on the other hand, has been correlated with decreased CREB activity, dendritic complexity, and synaptic density and is translocated during extra synaptic NMDAR stimulation [79].

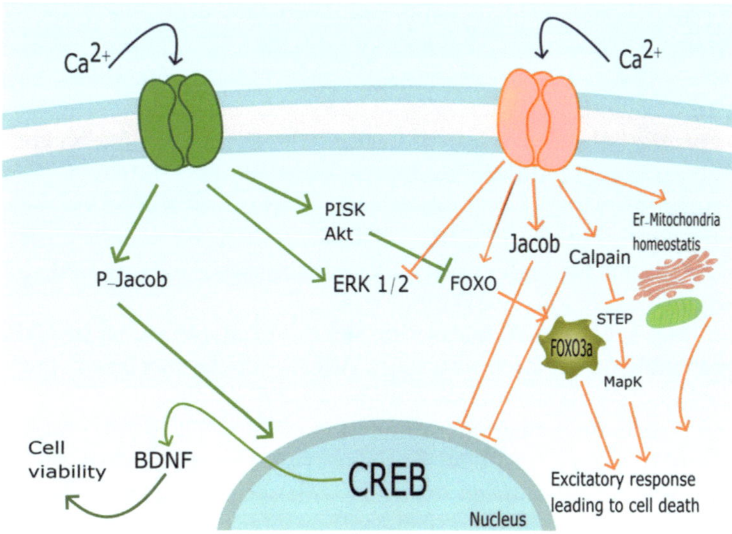

Figure 7.
Synaptic (green) and extrasynaptic (red) NMDAR signaling pathways. Synaptic NMDARs phosphorylate Jacob, activate ERK1/2, and promote CREB activation, enhancing BDNF expression, cell viability, and neuroprotection. Extrasynaptic NMDARs facilitate Jacob nuclear import, FOXO activation, calpain-mediated STEP activation, ER-mitochondrial disruption, and excitotoxicity, leading to cell death.

3.5.5 FoxO3a and ERK signaling

FoxO3a, a fork head transcription factor, influences neuronal function via pathways regulating oxidative stress, autophagy, apoptosis, and mitochondrial activity. FoxO3a modulation affects cognitive decline in AD, stroke, and Parkinson's disease. Increased extrasynaptic NMDAR activity translocate FoxO3a to the nucleus, promoting excitotoxic cell death. Synaptic NMDARs, however, restrict FoxO3a activity through Akt-mediated phosphorylation [71, 80]. Synaptic and extra synaptic NMDARs have opposite effects on the ERK1/2 pathway, which plays a role in neuroprotection mediated by NMDAR. Extra synaptic NMDAR stimulates Calpain, a calcium-dependent protease that is evoked by raised intracellular calcium levels, and a cascade of events lead to the cleavage of striatal enriched tyrosine phosphatase (STEP)61 into STEP33. Unlike STEP61, STEP33 is devoid of a regulatory domain and exhibits continuous activity, which can lead to the dephosphorylation and inactivation of proteins influencing synaptic function. Synaptic NMDAR activation leads to the reduced degeneration of STEP because of STEP61 ubiquitination and degradation, which is associated with ERK1/2 phosphorylation [81].

The ERK1/2 pathway activates CREB which has been linked to NMDAR-mediated neuroprotection. NMDARs play a bi-directional role in ERK regulation based on their localization i.e. synaptic or extra synaptic. Synaptic NMDARs activate ERK, whereas extra synaptic NMDARs deactivate it [82]. Thus, synaptic and extra synaptic NMDARs are mutually antagonistic compared to ERK signaling (**Figure 7**).

4. Therapeutic targets in Alzheimer's disease

The National Institute on Aging identifies two classes of FDA-approved drugs for AD treatment: cholinesterase inhibitors and memantine, an NMDAR antagonist [59].

Memantine reduces tau phosphorylation and prevents neuronal necrosis, impaired axonal transport, DNA damage, and neurite retraction [83]. Trodusquemine mitigates Aβ toxicity [84]. while Neramexane, another NMDAR antagonist, improves memory in animal models [85].

AD disrupts the balance between protective GluN2A-containing synaptic NMDARs and excitotoxic GluN2B-containing extrasynaptic NMDARs. Ifenprodil (a GluN2B antagonist) and D-cycloserine (a co-activator of NMDARs) together showed better protective effects against Aβ toxicity than either alone [86], Enhancing GluN2A activity alone through positive allosteric modulation (e.g., GNE-0723) also improved cognitive function in AD models [47],

These findings suggest that modulating synaptic and extrasynaptic NMDAR activity could be a viable AD treatment strategy. Altering co-agonist levels (glycine and D-serine) may also regulate NMDAR activity [19, 79].

Repetitive transcranial magnetic stimulation (rTMS) has shown promise in AD, Parkinson's, and schizophrenia. Low-frequency rTMS improves NMDAR levels, LTP, and spatial memory in Aβ-induced AD mice, with positive cognitive effects in human trials [56, 87]. Selenium-methionine (Se-Met) restores synaptic integrity by modulating Ca^{2+} influx via NMDARs, leading to improved cognitive function [88].

Table 3 below summarizes aforementioned evidence into Glutamate Modulation, NMDAR subunit targeting and Novel approaches.

Category	Therapy	Mechanism	Effect in AD models/ Humans	Reference
1. Glutamate Modulation	**Memantine** (FDA-approved)	Non-competitive NMDAR antagonist	Reduces tau phosphorylation, neuronal necrosis, axonal transport defects, DNA damage, neurite retraction	[59, 83]
	Neramexane	NMDAR antagonist (memantine derivative)	Improves memory and learning in animal AD models	[85]
	Trodusquemine	Indirect glutamate modulator via Aβ inhibition	Mitigates Aβ toxicity, reducing synaptic damage	[84]
2. NMDAR Subunit Targeting	**Ifenprodil**	Selective GluN2B subunit antagonist (extrasynaptic NMDAR)	Reduces excitotoxicity; enhances Aβ protection when combined with D-cycloserine	[86]
	D-cycloserine	Partial NMDAR co-agonist (at glycine site)	Enhances synaptic NMDAR function; synergistic neuroprotection with Ifenprodil	[86]
	GNE-0723	Positive allosteric modulator of GluN2A-containing NMDARs	Enhances synaptic NMDAR activity; improves cognitive function	[47]
	Glycine / D-serine modulation	Co-agonist level alteration to fine-tune NMDAR activity	May restore NMDAR homeostasis in AD brains	[19, 79, 89]
3. Novel Approaches	**rTMS** (Repetitive Transcranial Magnetic Stimulation)	Non-invasive brain stimulation; enhances NMDAR activity and LTP	Improves spatial memory, synaptic plasticity; positive human trial outcomes	[56, 87]

Category	Therapy	Mechanism	Effect in AD models/ Humans	Reference
	Selenium-methionine (Se-Met)	Regulates Ca^{2+} influx through NMDARs; antioxidant	Restores synaptic integrity; improves cognition in Aβ mouse models	[88]

Table 3.
Summary of therapeutic strategies in AD.

4.1 Biomarker-based monitoring in Alzheimer's disease: Key challenges and emerging approaches

4.1.1 Key challenges

Monitoring treatment efficacy in Alzheimer's disease (AD) using biomarkers remains a formidable challenge, despite significant advancements in their diagnostic utility. Currently established biomarkers—such as amyloid-β and tau; while useful for early and differential diagnosis, fall short in reliably tracking therapeutic response and disease progression, particularly in clinical trials that target amyloid-β pathways [90–94]. This underscores a critical limitation in their scope and sensitivity. Furthermore, a major gap exists in the availability of biomarkers that reflect non-amyloid and non-tau pathologies. Key pathological processes such as neuroinflammation, oxidative stress, lipid metabolism, vascular damage, and impaired protein clearance are underrepresented in current biomarker panels, yet they play essential roles in AD pathogenesis [90, 92–95].

Validation and standardization also pose significant barriers; Although novel biomarkers like neurofilament light (NfL), neurogranin, and YKL-40 show potential, they remain inadequately validated and lack standardized protocols across research centers. This hampers their utility in multi-center trials and clinical translation [92–94]. Additionally, there are practical challenges concerning biomarker accessibility. Cerebrospinal fluid (CSF)-based tests, while reliable, are invasive and less suited for routine clinical monitoring. Although blood-based biomarkers are a promising alternative, they are influenced by patient heterogeneity, blood-brain barrier permeability, and preanalytical variability—factors that complicate consistent measurement [93, 94].

4.1.2 Emerging solutions and approaches

To overcome these limitations, several innovative strategies are under exploration. One promising approach is the use of combination biomarker panels that integrate markers of neurodegeneration, synaptic function, and inflammation. These composite profiles can provide a more nuanced and comprehensive understanding of AD pathology, thus improving the accuracy of treatment monitoring [90, 92, 93, 95]. In parallel, digital and multimodal technologies, such as electroencephalography (EEG) and functional near-infrared spectroscopy (fNIRS), are being paired with fluid biomarkers to enable real-time tracking of cognitive changes and therapeutic impact [96]. This reflects a shift toward dynamic and personalized monitoring. Additionally, the integration of systems bioloy, where biomarker data is combined with cognitive assessments, clinical measures, and neuroimaging—holds promise for capturing disease heterogeneity and progression more effectively [92].

While biomarkers have revolutionized the diagnosis of AD, their role in monitoring treatment remains constrained by limited specificity, standardization, and practicality. Addressing these issues requires a multi-pronged strategy: expanding the biomarker repertoire beyond amyloid and tau, validating emerging candidates across diverse populations and centers, and embracing multimodal data integration. Such advances are essential for enabling precision medicine approaches in AD therapy.

5. Conclusion

In summary, glutamate is a foundation of CNS neurotransmission, acting as the main excitatory neurotransmitter that provides synaptic communication and facilitates such important processes as synaptic plasticity, learning, and memory. Glutamate levels are tightly regulated by neurons and glial cells to maintain effective signaling and protect neurons from excitotoxicity. The balance has to be maintained; even minor imbalances will have serious effects on brain health.

Glutamatergic signaling dysregulation has come to be increasingly acknowledged as a core contributor to a variety of neurological and neurodegenerative diseases. In Alzheimer's disease (AD), such disruption is especially marked. Exaggerated activation of glutamate receptors—particularly NMDA receptors—results in prolonged excitotoxicity, propelling neuronal damage and hastening cognitive deterioration. This situation is compounded by dysfunctional glutamate transporters, which are unable to effectively remove surplus extracellular glutamate, further fueling the neurotoxic milieu.

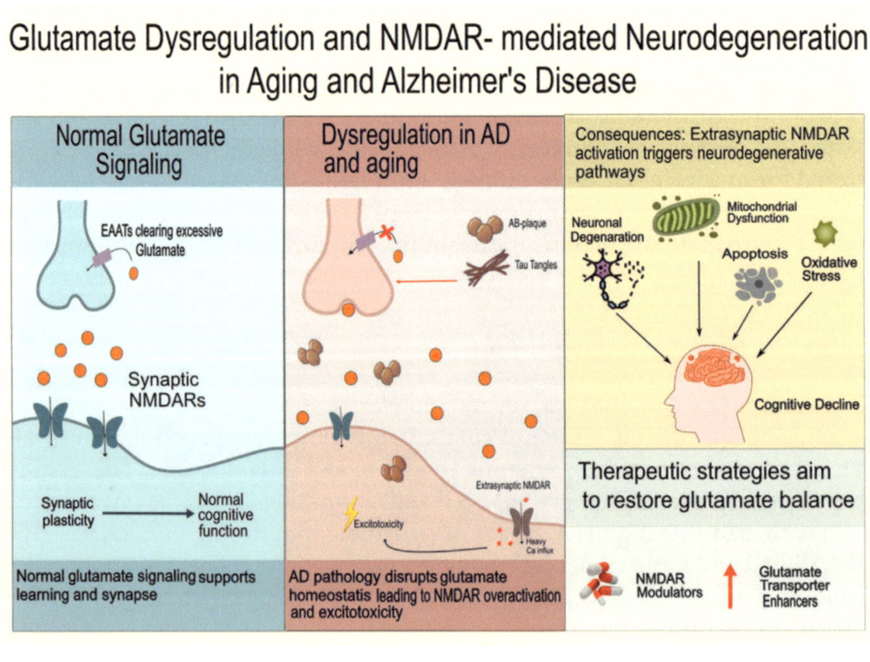

Figure 8.
This figure summarizes how disrupted glutamate clearance in Alzheimer's disease shifts NMDAR activation from synaptic to extrasynaptic sites, driving excitotoxicity and neurodegeneration, and highlights therapeutic approaches to restore glutamate balance.

Despite our great strides, a few knowledge gaps persist. The most important of these are the timing of NMDA receptor–targeted therapies, identification of a consistent biomarker to determine predisposition to excitotoxicity, and the optimal way to combine these interventions with current amyloid-β and tau-based treatments. Resolving these unknowns is important to transform our current understanding into effective, individualized therapeutic regimens.

Directions for the future need to center on the disentanglement of the complex regulation of glutamatergic signaling pathways and pathological derangement in disorders such as AD. Interventions that restore glutamate homeostasis, diminish receptor-mediated toxicity, and enhance synaptic resilience are extremely promising. With future advancements in research, addressing glutamatergic dysfunction may not just be able to slow disease progression but also provide a bridge to maintaining cognition and enhancing outcome for the persons with neurodegenerative disorders (**Figure 8**).

Conflict of interest

The authors declare no conflict of interest.

Author details

Ammarah Baig[1], Javeria Tanveer[2], Rukhsana Rubeen[3], Shazia Shakoor[4], Kanza Khan[2] and Kaneez Fatima-Shad[5]*

1 Aga Khan University, Karachi, Pakistan

2 Jinnah University for Women, Karachi, Pakistan

3 Dow University of Health and Sciences Karachi, Pakistan

4 Bahria University Medical and Dental College, Karachi, Pakistan

5 School of Life Sciences, University of Technology Sydney, Australia

*Address all correspondence to: ftmshad@gmail.com
and kaneez.fatima-shad@uts.edu.au

References

[1] Zhou Y, Danbolt NC. Glutamate as a neurotransmitter in the healthy brain. Journal of Neural Transmission. 2014;**121**(8):799-817

[2] Albrecht J, Sidoryk-Węgrzynowicz M, Zielińska M, Aschner M. Roles of glutamine in neurotransmission. Neuron Glia Biology. 2010;**6**(4):263-276

[3] Yelamanchi SD, Jayaram S, Thomas JK, Gundimeda S, Khan AA, Singhal A, et al. A pathway map of glutamate metabolism. Journal of Cell Communication and Signaling. 2015;**10**(1):69-75

[4] Willard SS, Koochekpour S. Glutamate, glutamate receptors, and downstream signaling pathways. International Journal of Biological Sciences. 2013;**9**(9):948-959

[5] Vandenberg RJ, Ryan RM. Mechanisms of glutamate transport. Physiological Reviews. 2013;**93**(4):1621-1657

[6] Schubert F, Gallinat J, Seifert F, Rinneberg H. Glutamate concentrations in human brain using single voxel proton magnetic resonance spectroscopy at 3 tesla. NeuroImage. 2004;**21**:1762-1771

[7] Boumezbeur F, Mason GF, de Graaf RA, al et. Altered brain mitochondrial metabolism in healthy aging as assessed by in vivo magnetic resonance spectroscopy. Journal of Cerebral Blood Flow and Metabolism. 2010;**30**(1):211-221

[8] Segovia G, Porras A, Del Arco A, Mora F. Glutamatergic neurotransmission in aging: A critical perspective. Mechanisms of Ageing and Development. 2001;**122**:1-29

[9] Zhang X, Liu H, Wu J, Zhang X, Liu M, Wang Y. Metabonomic alterations in hippocampus, temporal and prefrontal cortex with age in rats. Neurochemistry International. 2009;**54**:481-487

[10] Kaiser L, Schuff N, Cashdollar N, Weiner M. Age-related glutamate and glutamine concentration changes in normal human brain: 1H MR spectroscopy study at 4 T. Neurobiology of Aging. 2005;**26**:665-672

[11] Zahr N, Mayer D, Pfefferbaum A, Sullivan E. Low striatal glutamate levels underlie cognitive decline in the elderly: Evidence from in vivo molecular spectroscopy. Cerebral Cortex. 2008;**18**:2241-2250

[12] Chang L, Jiang C, Ernst T, al et. Effects of age and sex on brain glutamate and other metabolites. Magnetic Resonance Imaging. 2009;**27**:142-145

[13] Conway M. Alzheimer's disease: Targeting the glutamatergic system. Biogerontology. 2020;**13**:257-274

[14] Zhong W, Wu A, Berglund K, Gu X, Jiang M, Talati J, et al. Pathogenesis of sporadic Alzheimer's disease by deficiency of NMDA receptor subunit GluN3A. Alzheimer's & Dementia. 2021;**18**:222-239

[15] Yu SP, Jiang M, Shim S, Pourkhodadad S, Wei L. Extrasynaptic NMDA receptors in acute and chronic excitotoxicity: Implications for preventive treatments of ischemic stroke and late-onset alzheimer's disease. Molecular Neurodegeneration. 2023;**18**:43

[16] Ortiz-Sanz C, Balantzategi U, Quintela-López T, Ruiz A, Luchena C, Zuazo-Ibarra J, et al. Amyloid β /

PKC-dependent alterations in NMDA receptor composition are detected in early stages of Alzheimer's disease. Cell Death & Disease. 2022;**13**(3):1-12

[17] Dejakaisaya H, Kwan P, Jones N. Astrocyte and glutamate involvement in the pathogenesis of epilepsy in Alzheimer's disease. Epilepsia. 2021;**62**(7):1485-1493

[18] Zhang ZH et al. Selenium restores synaptic deficits by modulating NMDA receptors and Selenoprotein K in an Alzheimer's disease model. Antioxidants & Redox Signaling. 2021;**35**(11):863-884

[19] Bell K, Ducatenzeiler A, Ribeiro-da-Silva A, Duff K, Bennett D, Claudio CA. The amyloid pathology progresses in a neurotransmitter-specific manner. Neurobiology of Aging. 2006;**27**:1644-1657

[20] Ferrarese C, Begni B, Canevari C, Zoia C, Piolti R, Frigo M, et al. Glutamate uptake is decreased in platelets from Alzheimer's disease patients. Annals of Neurology. 2000;**47**:641-643

[21] Rodriguez-Lopez A, Torres-Paniagua A, Acero G, Díaz G, Gevorkian G. Increased TSPO expression, pyroglutamate-modified amyloid beta (AβN3(pE)) accumulation and transient clustering of microglia in the thalamus of Tg-SwDI mice. Journal of Neuroimmunology. 2023;**382**:578150-578150

[22] Walsh D, Selkoe D. Amyloid β-protein and beyond: The path forward in Alzheimer's disease. Current Opinion in Neurobiology. 2020;**61**:116-124

[23] Lee V, Goedert M, Trojanowski J. Neurodegenerative tauopathies. Annual Review of Neuroscience. 2001;**24**:1121-1159

[24] Dabir DV, Robinson MB, Swanson E, Zhang B, Trojanowski JQ, Lee VM, et al. Impaired glutamate transport in a mouse model of tau pathology in astrocytes. The Journal of Neuroscience. 2006;**26**:644-654

[25] Parkin GM, Udawela M, Gibbons A, Dean B. Glutamate transporters, EAAT1 and EAAT2, are potentially important in the pathophysiology and treatment of schizophrenia and affective disorders. WJP. 2018;**8**(2):51-63

[26] Wood OWG, Yeung JHY, Palpagama TH, Turner C, Waldvogel HJ, Faull RLM, et al. Upregulated excitatory amino acid transporter 1 (EAAT1) expression in the human medial temporal lobe in Alzheimer's disease. Neuroscience. 2025;**566**:87-96

[27] Todd AC, Hardingham GE. The regulation of astrocytic glutamate transporters in health and neurodegenerative diseases. IJMS. 2020;**21**(24):9607

[28] Zoia C, Cogliati T, Tagliabue E, Cavaletti G, Sala G, Galimberti G, et al. Glutamate transporters in platelets: EAAT1 decrease in aging and in Alzheimer's disease. Neurobiology of Aging. 2004;**25**(2):149-157

[29] Li S, Mallory M, Alford M, Tanaka S, Masliah E. Glutamate transporter alterations in Alzheimer disease are possibly associated with abnormal APP expression. Journal of Neuropathology and Experimental Neurology. 1997;**56**(8):901-911

[30] Simpson JE, Ince PG, Lace G, Forster G, Shaw PJ, Matthews F, et al. Astrocyte phenotype in relation to Alzheimer-type pathology in the ageing brain. Neurobiology of Aging. 2010;**31**(4):578-590

[31] Liu SY, Ma YL, Hsu WL, Lee E. P1-206: Pias1 Ser-503 phosphorylation-mediated Elk-1 Sumoylation promotes neuronal survival in APP/PS1 mice. Alzheimer's & Dementia. 2019;**15**(7S_Part_6):315-316. DOI: 10.1016/j.jalz.2019.06.761

[32] Li SJ, Ma MH, Li JM, Lu XY, Lu CB, Zhou SF, et al. CNTN1 aggravates neuroinflammation and triggers cognitive deficits in male mice by boosting crosstalk between microglia and astrocytes. Aging and Disease. 2023;**14**(5):1853

[33] Han X, Yang L, Du H, Sun Q, Wang X, Cong L, et al. Insulin attenuates beta-amyloid-associated insulin/Akt/EAAT signaling perturbations in human astrocytes. Cellular and Molecular Neurobiology. 2016;**36**(6):851-864

[34] Thai D. Excitatory amino acid transporter EAAT-2 in tangle-bearing neurons in Alzheimer's disease. Brain Pathology. 2002;**12**:405-411

[35] Tamagno E, Guglielmotto M, Vasciaveo V, Tabaton M. Oxidative stress and Beta amyloid in Alzheimer's disease. Which comes first: The chicken or the egg? Antioxidants. 2021;**10**(9):1479

[36] Hampel H, Hardy J, Blennow K, Chen C, Perry G, Kim S, et al. The amyloid-β pathway in Alzheimer's disease. Molecular Psychiatry. 2021;**26**(10):5481-5503

[37] Bruni A, Bernardi L, Gabelli C. From beta amyloid to altered proteostasis in Alzheimer's disease. Ageing Research Reviews. 2020;**64**:101126

[38] Srivastava A, Das B, Yao A, Yan R. Metabotropic glutamate receptors in Alzheimer's disease synaptic dysfunction: Therapeutic opportunities and Hope for the future. Journal of Alzheimer's Disease. 2020;**78**(4):1345-1361

[39] Onyango I, Jauregui G, Čarná M, Bennett J, Stokin G. Neuroinflammation in Alzheimer's disease. Biomedicine. 2021;**9**(5):524

[40] Liu Y, Si Z, Zou C, Mei X, Li X, Luo H, et al. Targeting neuroinflammation in Alzheimer's disease: From mechanisms to clinical applications. Neural Regeneration Research. 2023;**18**(4):708

[41] Jellinger K. Neuropathological assessment of the Alzheimer spectrum. Journal of Neural Transmission. 2020;**127**(9):1229-1256

[42] Goedert M et al. Tau protein and frontotemporal dementias. In: Frontotemporal Dementias. Cham, Switzerland: Springer; 2021

[43] Muralidar S, Ambi S, Sekaran S, Thirumalai D, Palaniappan B. Role of tau protein in Alzheimer's disease: The prime pathological player. International Journal of Biological Macromolecules. 2020;**163**:1599-1617

[44] Qu L, Sha S, Xing X, Wang T, Li Y, Zhang R, et al. DNA vaccines targeting amyloid-β oligomer ameliorate cognitive deficits of aged APP/PS1/tau triple-transgenic mouse models of Alzheimer's disease. Neural Regeneration Research. 2022;**17**(10):2305

[45] Hashem J, Hu M, Zhang J, Gao F, Chen C, Singh D. Astrocytic and microglial cells as the modulators of neuroinflammation in Alzheimer's disease. Journal of Neuroinflammation. 2022;**19**(1):206

[46] Traynelis SF et al. Glutamate receptor ion channels: Structure,

regulation, and function. Pharmacological Reviews. 2010;**62**(3):405-496

[47] Hanson JE et al. GluN2A NMDA receptor enhancement improves brain oscillations, synchrony, and cognitive functions in Dravet syndrome and Alzheimer's disease models. Cell Reports. 2020;**30**(2):381-396.e4

[48] Duguid IC. Presynaptic NMDA receptors: Are they dendritic receptors in disguise? Brain Research Bulletin. 2013;**93**:4-9

[49] Zhang Y et al. Dysfunction of NMDA receptors in Alzheimer's disease. Neurological Sciences. 2016;**37**:1039-1047

[50] Takai H et al. Distribution of N-methyl-d-aspartate receptors (NMDARs) in the developing rat brain. Experimental and Molecular Pathology. 2003;**75**(1):89-94

[51] Henson MA et al. Developmental regulation of the NMDA receptor subunits, NR3A and NR1, in human prefrontal cortex. Cerebral Cortex. 2008;**18**(11):2560-2573

[52] Lau CG et al. Regulation of NMDA receptor Ca^{2+} signalling and synaptic plasticity. Biochemical Society Transactions. 2009;**37**(6):1369-1374

[53] Müller T et al. Both NR2A and NR2B subunits of the NMDA receptor are critical for long-term potentiation and long-term depression in the lateral amygdala of horizontal slices of adult mice. Learning & Memory. 2009;**16**(6):395-405

[54] Parsons MP, Raymond LA. Extrasynaptic NMDA receptor involvement in central nervous system disorders. Neuron. 2014;**82**(2):279-293

[55] Talantova M et al. Correction to supporting information for Talantova et al., aβ induces astrocytic glutamate release, extrasynaptic NMDA receptor activation, and synaptic loss. Proceedings of the National Academy of Sciences. 2015;**112**(28):3751-3752

[56] Papouin T et al. Synaptic and extrasynaptic NMDA receptors are gated by different endogenous coagonists. Cell. 2012;**150**(3):633-646

[57] Bourne HR, Nicoll R. Molecular machines integrate coincident synaptic signals. Cell. 1993;**72**:65-75

[58] Nevian T, Sakmann B. Single spine Ca^{2+} signals evoked by coincident EPSPs and backpropagating action potentials in spiny stellate cells of layer 4 in the juvenile rat somatosensory barrel cortex. The Journal of Neuroscience. 2004;**24**(7):1689-1699

[59] Hetman M, Kharebava G. Survival signaling pathways activated by NMDA receptors. Current Topics in Medicinal Chemistry. 2006;**6**:787-799

[60] Holtmaat A, Svoboda K. Experience-dependent structural synaptic plasticity in the mammalian brain. Nature Reviews Neuroscience. 2009;**10**(9):647-658

[61] Higley MJ, Sabatini BL. Calcium signaling in dendritic spines. Cold Spring Harbor Perspectives in Biology. 2012;**4**(4):a005686-a005686

[62] Volianskis A et al. Long-term potentiation and the role of N -methyl- d -aspartate receptors. Brain Research. 2015;**1621**:5-16

[63] Wang R, Reddy P. Role of glutamate and NMDA receptors in Alzheimer's disease. Journal of Alzheimer's Disease. 2017;**57**(4):1041-1048

[64] Citri A, Malenka RC. Synaptic plasticity: Multiple forms, functions, and mechanisms. Neuropsychopharmacology. 2008;**33**(1):18-41

[65] Granger AJ, Raymond RA. Expression mechanisms underlying long-term potentiation: A postsynaptic view, 10 years on. Philosophical Transactions of the Royal Society B: Biological Sciences. 2014;**369**(1633):20130136

[66] Wolosker H. NMDA receptor regulation by D-serine: New findings and perspectives. Molecular Neurobiology. 2007;**36**(2):152-164

[67] Oliet SHR, Mothet JP. Regulation of N-methyl-d-aspartate receptors by astrocytic d-serine. Neuroscience. 2009;**158**(1):275-283

[68] Mothet JP et al. Time and space profiling of NMDA receptor co-agonist functions. Journal of Neurochemistry. 2015;**135**(2):210-225

[69] Südhof TC. The synaptic vesicle cycle. Annual Review of Neuroscience. 2004;**27**(1):509-547

[70] Rudy CC et al. The role of the tripartite glutamatergic synapse in the pathophysiology of Alzheimer's disease. Aging and Disease. 2015;**6**(2):131

[71] Pal MM. Glutamate: The master neurotransmitter and its implications in chronic stress and mood disorders. Frontiers in Human Neuroscience. 2021;**15**:722323

[72] Henneberger C et al. Long-term potentiation depends on release of d-serine from astrocytes. Nature. 2010;**463**(7278):232-236

[73] Ferreira IL et al. Amyloid Beta peptide 1-42 disturbs intracellular calcium homeostasis through activation of GluN2B-containing N-methyl-d-aspartate receptors in cortical cultures. Cell Calcium. 2012;**51**(2):95-106

[74] Soni N et al. GLT-1 transporter: An effective pharmacological target for various neurological disorders. Pharmacology Biochemistry and Behavior. 2014;**127**:70-81

[75] Mota SI et al. Dysfunctional synapse in Alzheimer's disease—A focus on NMDA receptors. Neuropharmacology. 2014;**76**:16-26

[76] Kamat PK et al. Okadaic acid-induced tau phosphorylation in rat brain: Role of NMDA receptor. Neuroscience. 2013;**238**:97-113

[77] Alberini CM. Transcription factors in long-term memory and synaptic plasticity. Physiological Reviews. 2009;**89**(1):121-145

[78] Du H et al. Cyclophilin D deficiency rescues aβ-impaired PKA/CREB signaling and alleviates synaptic degeneration. Biochimica et Biophysica Acta (BBA)-Molecular Basis of Disease. 2014;**1842**(12):2517-2527

[79] Dieterich DC et al. Caldendrin–Jacob: A protein liaison that couples NMDA receptor signalling to the nucleus. PLoS Biology. 2008;**6**(2):e34

[80] Qin W et al. Regulation of forkhead transcription factor FoxO3a contributes to calorie restriction-induced prevention of Alzheimer's disease-type amyloid neuropathology and spatial memory deterioration. Annals of the New York Academy of Sciences. 2008;**1147**(1):335-347

[81] Dick O, Bading H. Synaptic activity and nuclear calcium signaling protect hippocampal neurons from death signal-associated nuclear translocation

of FoxO3a induced by extrasynaptic N-methyl-d-aspartate receptors. Journal of Biological Chemistry. 2010;**285**(25):19354-19361

[82] Xu J et al. Extrasynaptic NMDA receptors couple preferentially to excitotoxicity via calpain-mediated cleavage of STEP. The Journal of Neuroscience. 2009;**29**(29):9330-9343

[83] Siddiqui AJ et al. Targeting NMDA receptor in Alzheimer's disease: Identifying novel inhibitors using computational approaches. Frontiers in Pharmacology. 2023;**14**:1208968

[84] Song M, Rauw G, Baker G, Kar S. Memantine protects rat cortical cultured neurons against beta-amyloid-induced toxicity by attenuating tau phosphorylation. European Journal of Neuroscience. 2008;**28**(10):1989-2002

[85] Zhang L et al. Tyrosine phosphatase PTP1B impairs presynaptic NMDA receptor-mediated plasticity in a mouse model of Alzheimer's disease. Neurobiology of Disease. 2021;**156**:105402

[86] Huang Y et al. Modulating the balance of synaptic and extrasynaptic NMDA receptors shows positive effects against amyloid-β-induced neurotoxicity. Journal of Alzheimer's Disease. 2017;**57**(3):885-897

[87] Tan T. Others. Low-frequency (1Hz) repetitive transcranial magnetic stimulation (rTMS) reverses Aβ1-42-mediated memory deficits in rats. Experimental Gerontology. 2013;**48**(8):786-794

[88] Anderkova L, Rektorova I. Cognitive effects of repetitive transcranial magnetic stimulation in patients with neurodegenerative diseases—Clinician's perspective. Journal of the Neurological Sciences. 2014;**339**(1-2):15-25

[89] Meunier C et al. Contribution of astroglial Cx43 hemichannels to the modulation of glutamatergic currents by D-serine in the mouse prefrontal cortex. The Journal of Neuroscience. 2017;**37**(37):9064-9075

[90] Park SA, Han SM, Kim CE. New fluid biomarkers tracking non-amyloid-β and non-tau pathology in Alzheimer's disease. Experimental & Molecular Medicine. 2020;**52**(4):556-568

[91] Pascoal TA, Aguzzoli CS, Lussier FZ, Crivelli L, Suemoto CK, Fortea J, et al. Insights into the use of biomarkers in clinical trials in Alzheimer's disease. eBioMedicine. 2024;**108**:105322

[92] Tarawneh R. Biomarkers: Our path towards a cure for Alzheimer disease. Biomarker Insights. 2020;**15**:117727192097636

[93] Molinuevo JL, Ayton S, Batrla R, Bednar MM, Bittner T, Cummings J, et al. Current state of Alzheimer's fluid biomarkers. Acta Neuropathologica. 2018;**136**(6):821-853

[94] Henriksen K, O'Bryant SE, Hampel H, Trojanowski JQ, Montine TJ, Jeromin A, et al. The future of blood-based biomarkers for Alzheimer's disease. Alzheimer's & Dementia. 2014;**10**(1):115-131

[95] Zetterberg H, Bendlin BB. Biomarkers for Alzheimer's disease—Preparing for a new era of disease-modifying therapies. Molecular Psychiatry. 2021;**26**(1):296-308

[96] Zhang Y, Zhang Y, Jiang Z, Xu M, Qing K. The effect of EEG and fNIRS in the digital assessment and digital therapy of Alzheimer's disease: A systematic review. Frontiers in Neuroscience. 2023;**17**:1269359

Chapter 3

Glutamate Dysregulation in Cingulated Cortices Is Associated with Autism Spectrum Disorder Traits

Carmen Jimenez-Espinoza, Francisco Marcano Serrano and José González-Mora

Abstract

Autism spectrum disorder (ASD) is a severe developmental syndrome that arises largely as a disorder of the neural systems. Despite unclear etiology, one of the most studied causes is the increase in the excitation/inhibition relationship in the sensory and social systems which may explain certain phenotypic expressions in ASD. Glutamate (Glu) is the most important excitatory neurotransmitter in mammals, and the excessive activation of once N-methyl-D-aspartate (NMDA) receptors leads to neuronal death. Crucially, in this study, the finding of elevated Glu concentration [12.10 ± 3.92 (mM) $^{*}p = 0.02$] by 1H-MRS in the anterior cingulate cortices (ACC) provides strong empirical support for increased arousal in ASD. The imbalance of Glu in cingulated cortices was correlated to dysfunction of social skills, attention switching/tolerance to change, attention to detail, communication, and imagination, (the five deficits present in ASD described in the Autism Quotient test), suggesting new therapeutic avenues.

Keywords: autism spectrum disorders, excitotoxicity, cingulated cortices, spectroscopy resonance magnetic, social skills, attention switching/tolerance to change, attention to detail, imagination, communication

1. Introduction

Autism spectrum disorder (ASD) is a severe developmental syndrome that arises largely as a disorder of neural systems in early childhood. Currently, the etiology remains unclear, and therapeutic options for ASD are limited; however, one of the most studied causes currently is the imbalance in the excitation/inhibition relationship in the sensory systems that can explain the extensive phenotypic variations in ASD, which are generally characterized by deficits in social reciprocity, communication, imagination, and restrictions interests and behaviors [1, 2]. Moreover, it might present secondary medical symptoms that include sleep and eating disorders, anxiety, depression, attention problems, aggressive behavior toward others or themselves, epilepsy, and gastrointestinal problems. Given this scenario, treating a person with ASD is a serious health problem for specialized medical care, not to mention the high costs they generate.

Through the different magnetic resonance techniques applied in research, many studies have been carried out to observe the involvement the glutamate (Glu) in people with ASD. However, currently, data referring to adults with ASD are scarce, given that most studies have been carried out in childhood, increasingly aggravating the lack of specific pharmacotherapies for adults. The specific pharmacotherapeutic approach in ASD is one of the main objectives of research studies, hence the need to delve deeper into the search for biomarkers that lead to the development of novel drugs for therapeutic application in the clinic. In this sense, the evidence suggests that an imbalance in glutamatergic metabolism and its products is linked to pathophysiological changes in ASD [3–12]. The interest in the different resonance magnetic modalities highlights specific brain areas such as the involvement of the ACC, and posterior cingulate cortex (PCC) in ASD symptoms, specifically magnetic resonance spectroscopy which relates cingulated cortices dysfunction to deficits in joint attention and social skills in ASD [13–21]. Increasing of these, neuropathology advances [22–27], structural MRI [28–32], fMRI [33–40], PET [41, 42], and SPECT [43, 44], including EEG-evoked potentials [45–48] indicate the cingulated cortices as one of the most affected areas of the brain responsible for the symptoms of the autism triad mainly [49].

Taking into account the plentiful evidence mentioned above, our objective is to study the role of Glu metabolism in the ACC and PCC, and its correlation with the five phenotypical characteristics as domains of interest (social, communication, imagination, attention to detail, and attention shifting/change tolerance), evaluated in the psychometric Autism Spectrum Quotient (AQ) test for adults, which we will describe later [2]. Here, we report an independent study of glutamate metabolism in the cingulated cortices in adults with ASD. A deeper follow-up investigation leads to larger when related to highlighted symptoms and/or severity within the AQ test for adults with ASD.

2. The brain metabolism

From the physiological point of view, the metabolism of the brain is made up of a wide variety of molecules, including peptides, neurotransmitters, enzymes, etc., interacting with water. All these molecules, due to their functions and activity, can maintain the physiological balance necessary for the healthy functioning of the brain. A very controlled balance, which represents 80% of the mass of the brain and (2–3) % of the body weight that receives 15% of the blood flow at rest (quote), it is also one of the organs with greater energy demand, which consumes 20% of the oxygen and 25% of the glucose ingested by the body [50]. All this neurometabolic exchange must be rapid and effective, precisely because the brain has few energy reserves and only receives them through the cerebral vascular system, which implies a correct supply of cerebral circulation through the circle of Willis [51, 52].

There is a group of biomolecules in the brain that are detected by proton magnetic resonance spectroscopy, we refer to neurotransmitters, defined as endogenous substances that act as chemical messengers transmitting signals, and that are normally released by neurons into the synaptic space where they exert their function on other neurons or other target cells through a synapse. Although neurotransmitters are related to their overall excitatory or inhibitory activity, some neurotransmitters can exert both excitatory and inhibitory effects depending on the type of receptors that are present.

There are other molecules that can be released from the same axon terminals as neurotransmitters, and they are known as endogenous neuromodulators [53] of the central nervous system (CNS), also known as neuropeptides, which can increase, prolong, inhibit, or limit the effect of the main neurotransmitter on the postsynaptic membrane, which acts through a system of second messengers [54]. It has also been pointed out that defects in the synthesis, release, or degradation of some neurotransmitters are involved in the pathogenesis of many neurological, muscular, and psychiatric diseases [55]. Evaluating the dynamics of neurotransmitters and neuromodulators in both health and neurological diseases is a challenge, precisely due to the lack of *in vivo* tools to monitor them with high spatiotemporal resolution and thus have a clear understanding of their functions within the nervous system.

2.1 Glutamate

Glutamate is an amino acid that has the four basic criteria to be considered a neurotransmitter. It is one of the most important neurotransmitters in our nervous system and it has a very high concentration. Recognized for functions such as a mediator of memory formation, the management of attention, or the regulation of emotions, in addition to intervening in 80% of all synapses necessary in processes such as neuroplasticity, learning, or movement. The physiological role of glutamate and its dysfunction has gained importance in neurology and psychiatry to the extent that knowledge has deepened about its metabolism, types of receptors, transporters, and homeostasis mechanisms, whose dysfunction can lead to neuronal death.

Additionally, glutamate and aspartate are the brain's dominant excitatory amino acids and constitute the main transmitters of pyramidal cells, the dominant neurons of the cortex where developmental changes occur capable of carrying out transient steps in the visual cortex and the hippocampus, especially during critical periods [56].

The glutamatergic system is distributed throughout the CNS, unlike other neurotransmission systems with more discrete metabolic pathways, which is why Glu is considered a general activator of the CNS [57, 58]. Under physiological conditions, endogenous Glu is one of the most abundant amino acids in our body and is the main excitatory neurotransmitter whose main purpose is to provide energy to the brain. However, exogenous Glu can be dangerous for our brain health in excessive concentrations, causing neurotoxicity. From a functional point of view, Glu acts as an "on switch" in nerve pathways and requires the neurotransmitter g-aminobutyric acid (GABA) as an "off switch" providing the necessary balance between these two neurotransmitters for at proper functioning of the CNS and essential for regulating cognition, learning, memory, and emotional behaviors. The imbalance between Glu excitation and GABA inhibition leads to hyperarousal of CNS related to ASD symptoms [59, 60].

2.1.1 Compartmentalization of glutamate in nervous system cells

One of the functional characteristics of glutamate is the establishment of compartmentalization in neurons and astrocytes. Within glutamatergic transmission, the release of gliotransmitters is an event that occurs by astrocytes through calcium waves [61, 62], where the elevation of intracellular calcium upon physiological neuronal stimulation is initiated by the activation of the mGluR5 receptor. This fact makes the difference in the vision of astrocytes as neuronal support cells to cells actively participating in neurotransmission and therefore in the processes mediated by neurotransmission [63, 64], glutamate itself being one of the gliotransmitters released [65–67].

This is an indication of the biochemical participation of glial cells in the glutamatergic system, also called the glutamate-glutamine cycle. Here, astrocytes express two key enzymes in glutamate metabolism that are not expressed in neurons and one enzyme that is not expressed in astrocytes but is expressed in neurons. One of the enzymes expressed in astrocytes but not in neurons is glutamate dehydrogenase (GD) [68], indicative of glutamate compartmentalization in the CNS. Thus, the glia-neuron glutamate-glutamine coupling mechanism demonstrates that the expression of the enzyme glutamine synthetase (GS) is glia-specific [69].

There is also another important compartmentalization establishment for Glu, we are referring to the synthesis of the neuromodulator *N*-acetyl-aspartyl-glutamate (NAAG), which has been the target of study in recent decades. This dipeptide is synthesized from *N*-acetyl-aspartate (NAA) and Glu by the enzyme NAA-synthase following the anabolic pathway, forming a reservoir of Glu that cannot be metabolized, and the NAAG produced is hydrolyzed, under the catabolic pathway by the NAAG enzyme-peptidase, which releases glutamate by activating the mGluR3 receptor, where its metabolic activity occurs by interconnecting neurons, astrocytes, and oligodendrocytes.

This dipeptide derivative of NAA and L-glutamate acts as a neurotransmitter and neuromodulator and is widely distributed in the CNS and peripheral in millimolar [mM] concentrations [70, 71]. Here, the establishment compartmentalization of Glu involves the participation of neurons, oligodendrocytes, and astrocytes where development an important metabolic activity develops known as the tri-cellular metabolism system [72]. This is the only metabolic cycle of amino acids in the brain known yet, that requires the three types of nervous cells. One of the main functions of NAAG is precisely the activation of glutamate (mGluRs) receptors that act as selective agonists of group II metabotropic receptors (mGluR, mGluR3) and involved the potential importance of metabotropic glutamate receptors, showing the neuromodulator NAAG a good candidate for elucidate the glutamatergic pathway ASD targeting. Considering that NAAG is distributed together with different neurotransmitters including Glu and GABA.

2.2 Autism spectrum quotient test (AQ)

The AQ is an instrument to measure the degree to which an adult with normal intelligence has the traits associated with the autism spectrum. Baron-Cohen and colleagues have described the adult test as a new self-assessment screening instrument to measure the degree to which an individual of normal intelligence displays autistic traits and was translated into Spanish by Betty Trabal, Editorial Amat, S.L., Barcelona, [73] with reasonable construct validity in that item that is intended to measure each one of the five domains of interest (social, communication, imagination, attention to detail, and attention shifting/change tolerance) showing moderate to high alpha coefficients.

To carry out this study, the AQ test was previously validated in an aleatory sample of adults with Spanish as their mother tongue [74], the Spanish version of the AQ has shown satisfactory levels of internal consistency and supports the use of the Spanish version of the AQ for the evaluation of ASD. In this sense, is considered a valuable instrument to quickly quantify where a given individual falls on the continuum from autism to normality.

3. Materials and methods

To further *understand* the role of the glutamatergic imbalance in the cingulated cortices and their relationship with the development of ASD symptoms related to psychometric test AQ scores, we conducted a clinical study of proton magnetic resonance spectroscopy (1H-MRS) to explore the cerebral glutamate levels in ACC and PCC, and determine its correlation with the five undergo change characteristics in ASD development (social skills, attention to detail, attention shifting/tolerance of change, communication, and imagination) compared to control subjects.

3.1 Population recruitment, demographic, and behavioral evaluations

3.1.1 Participants

We recruited 61 adult participants: Nineteen subjects with ASD (3 females; mean ± age SD: 20.58 ± 0.71 years, range: 17.8–30.9 years) and 42 typical developmental (TD) control subjects (25 females; 23.2 ± 0.71 years, 18.4–31.5 years) free of psychiatric or developmental disorders participated (see **Table 1**). The 61 participants were further divided into four subtypes (AQ1, AQ2, AQ3, and AQ4) according to the AQ test for adult's cause met the AQ test score cut-off criteria in all five characteristics domains. All participants with ASD were recruited through the research program through the faculty of Health Sciences. Dept. of Basic Medical Sciences of University of La Laguna (ULL), Tenerife, Spain. Potential participants were excluded if they had a comorbidity, psychiatric, or medical disorder that affects brain development (e.g., schizophrenia or psychosis), a history of head injury, or a genetic disorder associated with ASD, for example, tuberous sclerosis or fragile X syndrome [75]. The participants with ASD who suffered from anxiety or depressive disorders, gastrointestinal disorders, and muscular hypotonia were not excluded, given the high frequency of these comorbidities in ASD. In addition, based on participants' self-report, all participants were without previous medication at the time of the examination.

Informed written consent was obtained from all participants or from their legal guardians, as well as ethical approval for this study provided by the ethical standards and the Helsinki Declaration of 1964, revised in 2000 and approved by our local ethics committee. This study was approved by the Research Ethics and Animal Welfare Committee (CEIBA) (registration number: CEIBA2013–0056) of the University of La Laguna.

Additionally, participants were assessed and stratified into four subgroups according to established categories, empirically derived from Baron-Cohen & collaborators, AQ test scores, where the subgroup algorithm, which combines scores on the five domains of the AQ: Social skills, attention shifting/tolerance to change, attention to detail, communication, and imagination defined the cut-off threshold for producing reliable ASD subgroups [73]. This approach is consistent with previous publications on this sample, providing a description of participant characteristics [74].

The AQ test score for adult, included the five symptom domains and was divided into four subtypes, each with the following cutoff and meaning: AQ1 (0 to 10 points) = below average; AQ2 (11–21 points) = average values of the normal

Demographic characteristics	ASD (n = 19) mean (S.D.)	(TD) (n = 42) mean (S.D.)	Statistics p value
Gender (male/female)	16/3	16/25	P = 0.016
Age (years)	20.58 /0.71)	23.19 (0.71)	P = 0.049
AQ (0–50) points	33.84 (6.36)	11.67 (7.07)	P < 0.0001
Social skills	5.92 (2.54)	1.22 (0.61)	P < 0.0001
Attention switching/tolerance to change	6.81 (1.41)	3.49 (2.06)	P < 0.0001
Attention to detail	4.3 (1.91)	5.03 (2.3)	P < 0.0001
Communication	7.5 (1.75)	2.15 (1.63)	P < 0.0001
Imagination	5.9 (1.82)	2.22 (1.59)	P < 0.0001
Muscular hypotonia	14	0	P < 0.0001
Gastrointestinal disorders	17	0	P < 0.0001
Epilepsy	5	0	P < 0.0015
Familial hypothyroidism	15	0	P < 0.0001
Special education/transition to adult life	6	0	P < 0.0008
Elementary school	13	41	P < 0.0002
Middle school	6	41	P < 0.0008
High school	3	41	P < 0.008

*ASD (autism spectrum disorder), TD (Typical development). *p, 0.05 vs. controls; values for age and AQ are group mean ± standard deviation (range). AQ = Autism Quotient.*

Table 1.
Demographic data, neuropsychological, and physical measures.

population (female mean is 15 and male mean is 17); AQ3 (22–31 points) = above average; AQ4 (32–50 points) = very high index of autistic characteristics (Asperger syndrome or high-functioning autism has an average score of 35). Due to the differences in the results of the AQ test domains, we carried out a follow-up to evaluate the neurometabolic pattern of the four subtypes (AQ1, AQ2, AQ3, and AQ4) in the studied population, according to the implication of autistic characteristics. Considering the AQ1 subtype as a typical development control group (TD).

3.2 Proton magnetic resonance spectroscopy (1H-MRS) data acquisition

Proton magnetic resonance spectroscopy (1H-MRS) is a non-invasive imaging method that provides spectroscopic information that allows us to infer the metabolic cellular activity of the individual studied. 1H-MRS data were acquired using a 3 T Signa-HD MR scanner (GE Healthcare, Waukesha, WI, USA). T2-weighted images were used for positioning the volumes of interest (VOIs). The single voxel acquisition used a spin-echo sequence recorded within the following parameters: TE = 23 ms, TR = 1070 ms, NEX = 2, flip angle = 90°, and 256 acquisitions with the point-resolved spectroscopy (PRESS) technique. During data acquisition, the same experienced neuroradiologist, blind to the clinical data, placed the voxels $(2 \times 2 \times 2)\ cm^3$ at the ACC and PCC (See **Figure 1**) so careful to exclude contamination of signal from the

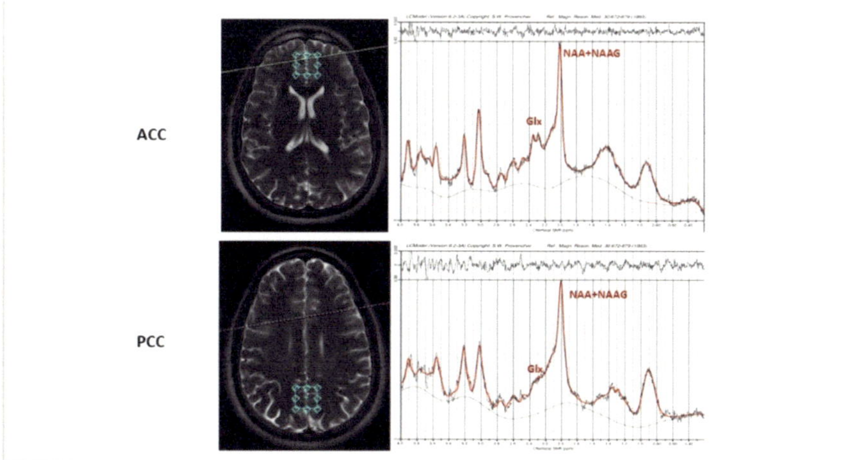

Figure 1.
Locations of the volume studied in the anterior (ACC) and posterior (PCC) cingulated cortices. The single voxel acquisition used a spin-echo sequence recorded within the following parameters: Echo time (TE) = 23 ms, repetition time (TR) = 1070 ms, 2 NEX, flip angle = 90, and 256 acquisitions with the point-resolved spectroscopy (PRESS) technique. During data acquisition, the same experienced neuroradiologist blinded the clinical data to place the voxels at interesting brain areas.

skull and subcutaneous fat. The 1H-MRS data sets collected showed the quantification of the absolute concentrations of brain metabolites, expressed in millimoles per kilogram of wet weight, involving the correction of many factors, such as the tissue composition of the voxel (relative amounts of cerebrospinal fluid and gray and white matter), the T1 and T2 relaxation times of the metabolites in the patient, the location of the voxels and their relationship with the electromagnetic properties of the coil, and any temporary variation in the scanner [76].

3.2.1 Automatic quantitation of localized in vivo *1H spectra*

LCModel is automatic (non-interactive) software version 6–1-0 (Stephen Provencher Incorporated, Oakville, Canada) [77] with no subjective input. Approximately maximum-likelihood estimates of the metabolite concentrations, phases, referencing shift, line shape, baseline, etc., and their uncertainties in the concentrations (Cramér-Rao lower bounds) are obtained [78]. The main metabolite resonances were limited for NAA, creatine and phosphocreatine, together abbreviated (Cr), choline-containing compounds phosphocholine, glycerophosphocholine, choline proper, and acetylcholine, together abbreviated (Cho), myo-inositol (mI), glutamate (Glu), glutamine (Gln), and the peak, "Glx," was for the sum of glutamate and glutamine [79]. One possible weakness of our method is the reliance on accurate suppression of the NAAG signal in the NAA scan, particularly the NAA signal in the NAAG scan (due to the higher concentration of NAA) [80]. An intense peak at 2 ppm is generally assigned to NAA (which is responsible for the greater part of the signal), but in this work, it was assumed to correspond to NAA + NAAG. Considered also, any small N-acetyl molecules in the brain will contribute to the peak, and moreover, small contributions from other N-acetyl species (e.g., N-acetyl-glutamate) could result in overestimation of the NAA and NAAG concentrations. Notwithstanding, the paradigm used here allowed us to resolve the NAAG peak with a %SD of <20% based on the reliability indicators or lower levels of Cramér–Rao. Each spectrum was reviewed to ensure an adequate signal-to-noise ratio, as well as the absence of artifacts which allowed us to define previously which were the best times TE/TR for the spectra obtained to show the highest number of metabolites.

The different metabolites were resolved using Cr as an internal reference according to LCModel, following standard clinical practice, because it is considered the most stable metabolite in cell tissue, [78]. Nor can the ratios of a metabolite represent all possible differences, if a single specific denominator is used (as is the case for creatine), if the signals recorded in all subjects were obtained in the same scanner unit and using the same protocol. Therefore, the excellent reproducibility for each metabolite allows us to quantify their absolute concentration in the ACC and PCC (see **Table 2**), and consequently to observe the different alterations in ASD (see **Figure 2**).

Anteriorly, studies have also used the LCModel in Ref. to disorders in epilepsy, [81–83] multiple sclerosis, [84–86] tumors, [87, 88] Alzheimer's disease, [89, 90] and other pathologies, [91–95] including the identification and quantitation of unusual metabolites, increasing the robustness of the results.

Brain area [mM]	ASD (n = 19) mean (S.D.)	TD (n = 42) mean (S.D.)	Statistics	P value
Anterior cingulate cortex				
NAA + NAAG	9.78 (0.49)	10.44 (0.29)		*p = 0.02
NAA	9.37 (1.36)	9.91 (0.68)	n.s.	
Glx(Glu+Gln)	16.10 (6.87)	15.19 (9.02)	n.s.	
Glu	12.10 (3.92)	10.54 (5.64)		*p = 0.02
GPC+PCh	2.08 (0.14)	2.08 (0.13)	n.s.	
Cr+PCr	6.98 (1.56)	7.40 (1.87)	n.s.	
mI	5.40 (0.78)	5.25 (0.27)	n.s.	
Posterior cingulate cortex				
NAA + NAAG	10.80 (0.86)	11.02 (0.68)	n.s.	
NAA	10.47 (1.39)	10.68 (0.20)	n.s.	
Glx(Glu+Gln)	13.87 (4.09)	14.08 (2.15)	n.s.	
Glu	10.22 (3.19)	10.71 (2.06)	n.s.	
GPC+PCh	1.55 (0.44)	1.61 (0.38)	n.s.	
Cr+PCr	6.72 (0.90)	6.99 (0.42)	n.s.	
mI	4.98 (0.68)	5.13 (1.94)	n.s.	

*The different metabolites concentrations detectable in ASD vs. TD, N-acetyl-aspartate (NAA), N-acetyl-aspartate + N-acetylaspartyl-glutamate (NAA + NAAG), glutamate+ glutamine Glx = (Glu + Gln), glutamate (Glu), creatine (PCr), choline (PCG + PCh), and myo-inositol (mI). Brain areas = anterior cingulate cortex (ACC) and posterior cingulate cortex (PCC). values for metabolites' absolute concentration are group mean ± standard deviation (range). *p < 0.05 considered significantly different, while n.s. represents non-significant results.*

Table 2.
Absolute metabolic concentrations detected by 1H-MRS.

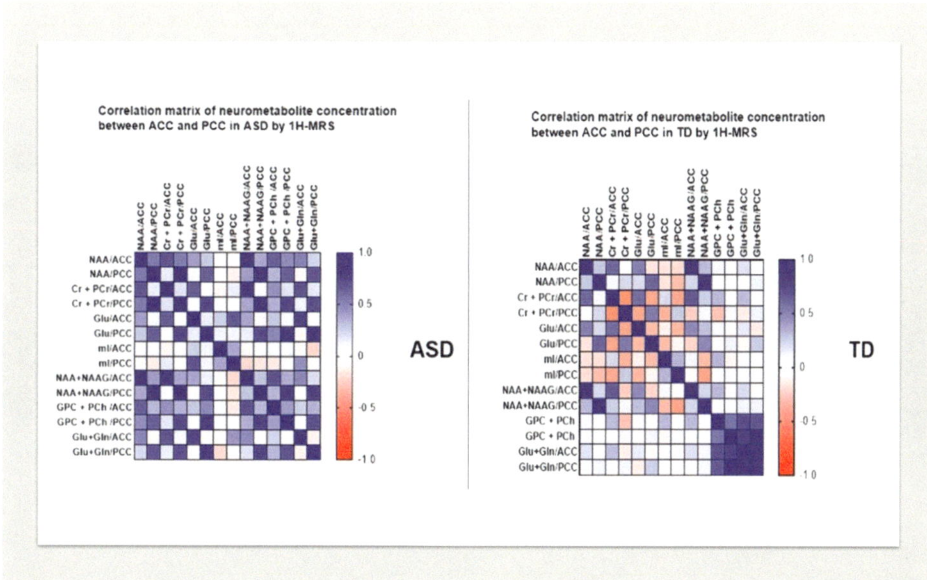

Figure 2.
The correlation matrix was used as a statistical technique to evaluate the relationship between two variables in metabolites' absolute concentrations set present in ACC and PCC, represented by values for N-acetyl aspartyl-glutamate (NAA + NAAG), glutamate + glutamine (Glx = Glu + Gln), glutamate (Glu), creatine (Cr + PCr), N-acetyl-aspartate (NAA), choline (GPC + PCh), and myo-inositol (mI) in ASD (n = 19) vs. TD (42). In this sense, we can summarize a large amount of data to identify patterns. Every cell contains a correlation coefficient, where 1 is considered a strong relationship between variables, 0 is a neutral relationship, and −1 is a not strong relationship. Above, the observed metabolic pattern is evidence of differences between subjects with or without autism. ($p < 0.05$) considers statistical significance.*

4. Results

4.1 Demographic characteristics data

Following our objective of characterizing the glutamate dysfunctions in adult subjects with ASD by quantifying (1) glutamate levels in the anterior and posterior cingulate cortex using proton magnetic resonance spectroscopy and, (2) its correlation with the AQ test on their different domains, of characteristics of ASD compared to the TD group presented in materials and method section. The ASD group differed significantly from the TD in the total AQ, which prompted us to use this psychometric test to correlate the Glu concentrations with each domain evaluated in the test.

4.2 Cingulate cortices neuro metabolites pattern in ASD

The 1H-MRS results showed an overall increase in Glu concentration in adults with ASD, which was only observed in ACC. This suggests that functional changes in Glu concentration could reflect an adaptation to previous glutamatergic dysfunctions rather than being key to the pathophysiology of ASD (see **Figure 3**).

However, when we diversified the population using the AQ test, a pattern was observed in the variation of Glu concentration linked to the severity of autistic

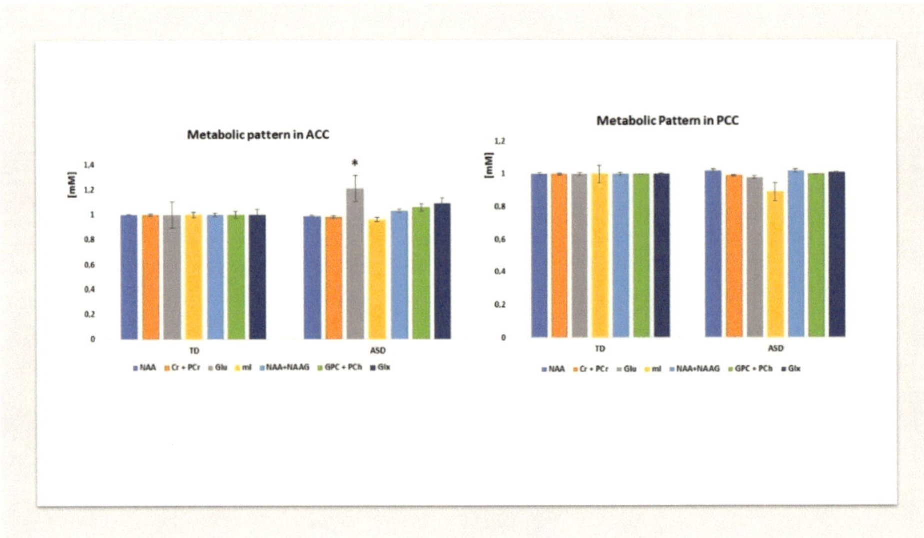

Figure 3.
*Normalized data metabolic variability of the different metabolites present in ACC and PCC in the ASD group (n = 19) and the TD group (n = 42), allows bias problems to be minimized. Glutamate is significantly elevated in the ACC, revealing a dysfunction pattern in excitatory/inhibitory metabolism in ACC patients with autism. (*p < 0.05) considers statistical significance.*

characteristics, evidencing the commitment of this neurotransmitter in the cingulated cortices. The compartmentalization of Glu with NAAG (see the introduction section) is also observed in ACC indicating a marked difference with PCC, which marks an important finding linked to ASD syndrome. (see **Figure 4**).

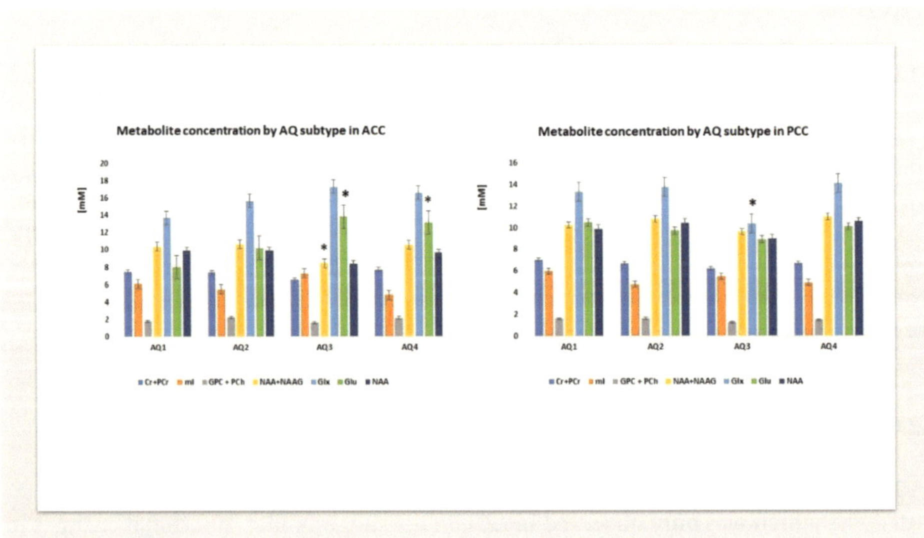

Figure 4.
*Pattern of variability of neurometabolites present in the cingulate cortices, when the ASD and TD groups were stratified into the AQ groups (AQ1, AQ2, AQ3, and AQ4), according to autistic characteristics. Graphic representation of the metabolic differentiation pattern and symptoms' severity between ACC and PCC. (*p < 0.05) considered significantly different.*

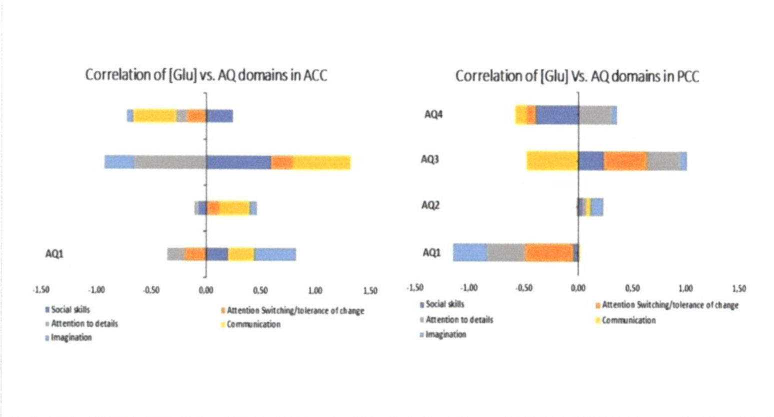

Figure 5.
*Graph of correlation pattern Pearson's coefficient of [Glu] concentration present in ACC and PCC, and the different autistic characteristics represented by AQ2, AQ3, and AQ4 groups with the AQ1 group taken as a reference or control of healthy AQ index, which can be used as a marker of the severity of symptoms in ACC and PCC. *$p < 0.05$ considered significantly different.*

4.3 Correlation of Glu with the autistic characteristics evaluated within the AQ

Here, interesting results were observed regarding Glu's commitment to each one of the five domains of interest (social, communication, imagination, attention to detail, and attention shifting/tolerance to change), suggesting how much it affects TD and the ASD group. Observing a direct correlation between Glu concentration and social skills, communication, and imagination in the AQ1 group (autistic characteristics below average). In contrast to the AQ4 group (very high index of autistic characteristics), where this direct correlation was observed with social skills only. However, the AQ3 group (above average), showed a direct correlation to social skills, attention switching/tolerance of change, and communication in ACC (see **Figure 5**). Suggest a broad interpretation of the effect caused by Glu dysfunction on the development of autistic triad mainly characteristics.

However, the results obtained in the PCC reflect that [Glu] concentration is directly correlated only with communication in the AQ1 group. Compared to the AQ4 group, which correlates directly with attention to detail and imagination. However, the AQ3 group shows a direct correlation with social skills, imagination, attention to detail, and attention shifting/tolerance to change, highlighting the biggest compromising of Glu dysfunction in this group.

One of the biggest concerns in children with autism is the development of speech or communication. This leads us to consider the importance of Glu dysfunction in PCC for groups AQ3 and AQ4 where autistic characteristics are more exacerbated, and its correlation with the development of communication.

5. Discussion

Herein, we presented evidence demonstrating a potential connection of ASD with glutamatergic dysfunction. We focused specifically on biochemical links, between ACC and PCC, and its functional connectivity.

The glutamatergic pathways in the brain are extensive. Glutamate is excreted into the synaptic cleft by the process of exocytosis or glutamatergic neurotransmission which involves processes of glial reuptake, presynaptic reuptake, AMPA agonism, NMDA agonism, and Kainate and Quisqualate receptor agonism.

In this 1H-MRS study, the finding of a significant increase in Glu concentration in the ACC, observed in adults with ASD, is in line with previous studies that reflect an imbalance of excitation/inhibition in the children and young brain [96–98], and support the hypothesis of excitatory/inhibitory imbalance in ASD.

The excitotoxicity induced by an increase in the level of Glu in the brain can have pathological consequences, due to the deregulation of intracellular Ca^{2+} concentrations. This delicate balance between the mechanisms that allow the entry of physiological Ca^{2+} and those that can limit the intracellular excess to avoid neurodegenerative processes are the ones that determine the loss of neuronal viability [99]. This statement allows us to conjecture, that this significant increase in glutamate levels in the ACC would be a possible cause of disorder within the autism spectrum, either due to deregulation of intracellular Ca^{2+} and/or, due to neurotoxicity due to excessive activation of NMDA receptors. Since they are the most permeable to calcium Ca^{2+}, and act cooperatively with AMPA-kainate-type receptors, fundamentally permeable to sodium [100].

Other studies have found atypical undergrowth of auditory and visual networks which was associated with the severity of autistic core socio-communication symptoms, that of the visual network was correlated with the severity of restricted and repetitive behaviors in ASD adults [101].

In this sense, in deregulation due to excess glutamate, there is a risk of losing cognitive capacity and even cell death, even in adults. Therefore, due to the role that glutamate has in various neurodegenerative pathologies, it results in an important – although also complex – pharmacological target. In this study, it was observed how an excess of glutamate in the cingulate cortex intervenes in the cognitive development of adult subjects with autism from childhood, when comparing them with neurotypical subjects. From the cognitive impairment that affects the functioning of functions such as attention, imagination, communication, and detail, as well as tolerance to change, to the main and most studied to date in the autistic condition - social skills - as seen in **Figure 5**.

An important milestone is the finding presented here of the metabolic deregulation of Glu, reported in the cingulate cortices, that justifies the hypofunction of the principal networks: The salience network (SAN), the default network (DMN), and the frontotemporal visual networks; as well as the motor skills which confirm the functional and neurochemical differences between ACC and PCC in subjects with ASD [102]. In addition to this, the dendritic complexity of the PCC is much lower than that present in the ACC, as other authors have shown [103], which would explain the metabolic differences between both regions in ASD and that are balanced in neurotypical subjects.

6. Conclusions

- The effects of excess glutamate in the **ACC** in subjects with ASD are directly correlated with the three central characteristics within the autism spectrum.

- The study of Glu receptors is ambitious in allowing greater knowledge of the functioning of the nervous system in people with ASD, which will open the doors for the development of more effective therapeutic strategies based on the regulation of glutamatergic neurotransmission.

- Currently, numerous NMDA receptor antagonists have been synthesized to reduce the entry of cal2+ through the targets of the AMPA-Kainate and NMDA receptors and thus reduce the excitotoxic effect of glutamate in the brain, but their clinical development is limited and has been hampered by the appearance of important adverse effects that would make its implementation in therapeutics difficult.

- Not surprisingly, drugs developed through animal models for ASD have not had enough success in human trials to justify their use in the clinic, and therefore there may be little enthusiasm for investing in Glu-regulating drugs as a possible therapeutic approach. Perhaps it is time to consider the investments that will bring this knowledge to the clinic.

Acknowledgements

Mainly we want to thank the Roviralta Foundation (Barcelona, Spain) for financing this pioneering project in the Canary Islands. As well as all the people who voluntarily participated in this study, technical and medical staff from the Canary Islands University Hospital (HUC), and the Magnetic Resonance Service for Biomedical Research (SEGAI). To the associations (APANATE, ASPERTEN, and ALDIS) that represent and serve the population with ASD in Tenerife, Canary Islands, Spain; for giving me your trust and support and for making all the years of effort worth it. I would like to add it under acknowledgments as funding ("Examination of GABA/glutamate neurotransmitters and functional connectivity in cognitive inhibition tasks. PID2021-126172NB-I00").

Conflict of interest

The authors declare no conflict of interest.

Author details

Carmen Jimenez-Espinoza*, Francisco Marcano Serrano and José González-Mora
Laboratory Neurochemistry and Neuroimages, Physiology Section, Faculty of Health Sciences, Department of Basic Medical Sciences, University of La Laguna, Tenerife, Spain

*Address all correspondence to: carmen.jimenez.87@ull.edu.es

References

[1] Roehr B. American psychiatric association explains DSM-5. BMJ. 2013;**6**:346

[2] Baron-Cohen S, Wheelwright S, Skinner R, Martin J, Clubley E. The autism-spectrum quotient (AQ): Evidence from Asperger syndrome/high-functioning autism, males and females, scientists, and mathematicians. Journal of Autism and Developmental Disorders. 2001;**31**:603

[3] Rubenstein JL, Merzenich MM. Model of autism: Increased ratio of excitation/inhibition in key neural systems. Genes, Brain and Behavior. 2003;**2**(5):255-267

[4] Oblak A, Gibbs TT, Blatt G. Decreased GABAA receptors and benzodiazepine binding sites in the anterior cingulate cortex in autism. Autism Research. 2009;**2**(4):205-219

[5] Pizzarelli R, Cherubini E. Alterations of GABAergic signaling in autism spectrum disorders. Neural Plasticity. 2011;**2011**:297153

[6] Galineau L, Arlicot N, Dupont AC, Briend F, Houy-Durand E, Tauber C, et al. Glutamatergic synapse in autism: A complex story for a complex disorder. Molecular Psychiatry. 2023;**28**(2):801-809

[7] Briend F, Barantin L, Cléry H, Cottier JP, Bonnet-Brilhault F, Houy-Durand E, et al. Glutamate levels of the right and left anterior cingulate cortex in autistics adults. Progress in Neuro-Psychopharmacology and Biological Psychiatry. 2023;**30**(126):110801

[8] Libero LE, Reid MA, White DM, Salibi N, Lahti AC, Kana RK. Biochemistry of the cingulate cortex in autism: An MR spectroscopy study. Autism Research. 2016;**9**(6):643-657

[9] Montanari M, Martella G, Bonsi P, Meringolo M. Autism spectrum disorder: Focus on glutamatergic neurotransmission. International Journal of Molecular Sciences. 2022;**23**(7):3861

[10] Chakraborty P, Dey A, Gopalakrishnan AV, Swati K, Ojha S, Prakash A, et al. Glutamatergic neurotransmission: A potential pharmacotherapeutic target for the treatment of cognitive disorders. Ageing Research Reviews. 2023;**5**:101838

[11] Oya M, Matsuoka K, Kubota M, Fujino J, Tei S, Takahata K, et al. Increased glutamate and glutamine levels and their relationship to astrocytes and dopaminergic transmissions in the brains of adults with autism. Scientific Reports. 2023;**13**(1):11655

[12] Varfolomeev S, Bykov V, Tsybenova S. Kinetic model of the glutamate neuron-astrocytic system. N-acetylaspartylglutamate and glutamate carboxypeptidase. ChemRxiv. 2023. DOI: 10.26434/chemrxiv-2023-7r957

[13] Fujii E, Mori K, Miyazaki M, Hashimoto T, Harada M, Kagami S. Function of the frontal lobe in autistic individuals: A proton magnetic resonance spectroscopic study. The Journal of Medical Investigation. 2010;**57**(1, 2):35-44

[14] Levitt JG, O'Neill J, Blanton RE, Smalley S, Fadale D, McCracken JT, et al. Proton magnetic resonance spectroscopic imaging of the brain in childhood autism. Biological Psychiatry. 2003;**54**(12):1355-1366

[15] Oner O, Devrimci-Ozguven H, Oktem F, Yagmurlu B, Baskak B, Munir KM. Proton MR spectroscopy: Higher right anterior cingulate N-acetylaspartate/choline ratio in Asperger syndrome compared with healthy controls. American Journal of Neuroradiology. 2007;**28**(8):1494-1498

[16] Bernardi S, Anagnostou E, Shen J, Kolevzon A, Buxbaum JD, Hollander E, et al. *In vivo* 1H-magnetic resonance spectroscopy study of the attentional networks in autism. Brain Research. 2011;**22**(1380):198-205

[17] Gabis L, Huang W, Azizian A, DeVincent C, Tudorica A, Kesner-Baruch Y, et al. 1H-magnetic resonance spectroscopy markers of cognitive and language ability in clinical subtypes of autism spectrum disorders. Journal of Child Neurology. 2008;**23**(7):766-774

[18] Mundy P. Annotation: The neural basis of social impairments in autism: The role of the dorsal medial-frontal cortex and anterior cingulate system. Journal of Child Psychology and Psychiatry. 2003;**44**(6):793-809

[19] Ito H, Mori K, Harada M, Hisaoka S, Toda Y, Mori T, et al. A proton magnetic resonance spectroscopic study in autism spectrum disorder using a 3-tesla clinical magnetic resonance imaging (MRI) system: The anterior cingulate cortex and the left cerebellum. Journal of Child Neurology. 2017;**32**(8):731-739

[20] Du Y, Chen L, Yan MC, Wang YL, Zhong XL, Xv CX, et al. Neurometabolite levels in the brains of patients with autism spectrum disorders: A meta-analysis of proton magnetic resonance spectroscopy studies (N= 1501). Molecular Psychiatry. 2023;**28**:1-2

[21] Gudmundson AT, Koo A, Virovka A, Amirault AL, Soo M, Cho JH, et al. Meta-analysis and open-source database for *in vivo* brain magnetic resonance spectroscopy in health and disease. Analytical Biochemistry. 2023;**1**(676):115227

[22] Vogt BA. Regions and subregions of the cingulate cortex. In: Cingulate Neurobiology and Disease. Vol. 4 (1). Oxford: Oxford Academic; 2009. p. 31

[23] Hadders-Algra M. Emerging signs of autism spectrum disorder in infancy: Putative neural substrate. Developmental Medicine & Child Neurology. 2022;**64**(11):1344-1350

[24] Xiong Y, Chen J, Li Y. Microglia and astrocytes underlie neuroinflammation and synaptic susceptibility in autism spectrum disorder. Frontiers in Neuroscience. 2023;**20**(17):1125428

[25] Ecker C, Schmeisser MJ, Loth E, Murphy DG. Neuroanatomy and neuropathology of autism spectrum disorder in humans. Translational Anatomy and Cell Biology of Autism Spectrum Disorder. 2017;**224**:27-48

[26] Yenkoyan K, Grigoryan A, Fereshetyan K, Yepremyan D. Advances in understanding the pathophysiology of autism spectrum disorders. Behavioural Brain Research. 2017;**28**(331):92-101

[27] Fetit R, Hillary RF, Price DJ, Lawrie SM. The neuropathology of autism: A systematic review of post-mortem studies of autism and related disorders. Neuroscience & Biobehavioral Reviews. 2021;**1**(129):35-62

[28] Pagnozzi AM, Conti E, Calderoni S, Fripp J, Rose SE. A systematic review of structural MRI biomarkers in autism spectrum disorder: A machine learning perspective. International Journal of Developmental Neuroscience. 2018;**1**(71):68-82

[29] Stigler KA, McDonald BC, Anand A, Saykin AJ, McDougle CJ. Structural and functional magnetic resonance imaging of autism spectrum disorders. Brain Research. 2011;**22**(1380):146-161

[30] Katuwal GJ, Cahill ND, Baum SA, Michael AM. The predictive power of structural MRI in autism diagnosis. In: 2015 37th Annual International Conference of the Ieee Engineering in Medicine and Biology Society (EMBC). Milan, Italy: IEEE; 2015. pp. 4270-4273. DOI: 10.1109/EMBC.2015.7319338

[31] Ali MT, ElNakieb Y, Elnakib A, Shalaby A, Mahmoud A, Ghazal M, et al. The role of structure MRI in diagnosing autism. Diagnostics. 2022;**12**(1):165

[32] Dekhil O, Ali M, Haweel R, Elnakib Y, Ghazal M, Hajjdiab H, et al. A comprehensive framework for differentiating autism spectrum disorder from neurotypicals by fusing structural MRI and resting state functional MRI. Seminars in Pediatric Neurology. 2020;**34**:100805

[33] Philip RC, Dauvermann MR, Whalley HC, Baynham K, Lawrie SM, Stanfield AC. A systematic review and meta-analysis of the fMRI investigation of autism spectrum disorders. Neuroscience & Biobehavioral Reviews. 2012;**36**(2):901-942

[34] Silani G, Bird G, Brindley R, Singer T, Frith C, Frith U. Levels of emotional awareness and autism: An fMRI study. Social Neuroscience. 2008;**3**(2):97-112

[35] Koshino H, Carpenter PA, Minshew NJ, Cherkassky VL, Keller TA, Just MA. Functional connectivity in an fMRI working memory task in high-functioning autism. NeuroImage. 2005;**24**(3):810-821

[36] Pierce K. Early functional brain development in autism and the promise of sleep fMRI. Brain Research. 2011;**22**(1380):162-174

[37] Hull JV, Dokovna LB, Jacokes ZJ, Torgerson CM, Irimia A, Van Horn JD. Resting-state functional connectivity in autism spectrum disorders: A review. Frontiers in Psychiatry. 2017;**4**(7):205

[38] Liu M, Li B, Hu D. Autism spectrum disorder studies using fMRI data and machine learning: A review. Frontiers in Neuroscience. 2021;**15**(15):697870

[39] Koshino H, Kana RK, Keller TA, Cherkassky VL, Minshew NJ, Just MA. fMRI investigation of working memory for faces in autism: Visual coding and underconnectivity with frontal areas. Cerebral Cortex. 2008;**18**(2):289-300

[40] Karavallil Achuthan S, Coburn KL, Beckerson ME, Kana RK. Amplitude of low frequency fluctuations during resting state fMRI in autistic children. Autism Research. 2023;**16**(1):84-98

[41] Nakamura K, Sekine Y, Ouchi Y, Tsujii M, Yoshikawa E, Futatsubashi M, et al. Brain serotonin and dopamine transporter bindings in adults with high-functioning autism. Archives of General Psychiatry. 2010;**67**(1):59-68

[42] Andersson M, Tangen Ä, Farde L, Bölte S, Halldin C, Borg J, et al. Serotonin transporter availability in adults with autism—A positron emission tomography study. Molecular Psychiatry. 2021;**26**(5):1647-1658

[43] Makkonen I, Riikonen R, Kokki H, Airaksinen MM, Kuikka JT. Serotonin and dopamine transporter binding in children with autism determined by SPECT. Developmental Medicine & Child Neurology. 2008;**50**(8):593-597

[44] Oblak A, Gibbs TT, Blatt GJ. Reduced serotonin receptor subtypes in a

limbic and a neocortical region in autism. Autism Research. 2013;**6**(6):571-583

[45] Brittenham C, Gordon J, Zemon VM, Siper PM. Objective frequency analysis of transient visual evoked potentials in autistic children. Autism Research. 2022;**15**(3):464-480

[46] Trenado C, González-Ramírez A, Lizárraga-Cortés V, Pedroarena Leal N, Manjarrez E, Ruge D. The potential of trial-by-trial variabilities of ongoing-EEG, evoked potentials, event related potentials and fMRI as diagnostic markers for neuropsychiatric disorders. Frontiers in Neuroscience. 2019;**17**(12):850

[47] Black MH, Chen NT, Iyer KK, Lipp OV, Bölte S, Falkmer M, et al. Mechanisms of facial emotion recognition in autism spectrum disorders: Insights from eye tracking and electroencephalography. Neuroscience & Biobehavioral Reviews. 2017;**1**(80):488-515

[48] Aykan S, Gürses E, Tokgöz-Yılmaz S, Kalaycıoğlu C. Auditory processing differences correlate with autistic traits in males. Frontiers in Human Neuroscience. 2020;**7**(14):584704

[49] Cashin A, Barker P. The triad of impairment in autism revisited. Journal of Child and Adolescent Psychiatric Nursing. 2009;**22**(4):189-193

[50] Guyton AC, Hall JE. Tratado de fisiologia médica. 12aed ed. Madrid-España: El Seiver; 2011. p. 432

[51] Vrselja Z, Brkic H, Mrdenovic S, Radic R, Curic G. Function of circle of Willis. Journal of Cerebral Blood Flow & Metabolism. 2014;**34**(4):578-584

[52] Rosner J, Reddy V, Lui F. Neuroanatomy, Circle of Willis. Treasure Island (FL): StatPearls Publishing; 2018

[53] Curtis H. Invitación a la Biología. Editorial Médica Panamericana; San Juan, Puerto Rico; 2006

[54] Snell RS. Los núcleos de los nervios craneales, sus conexiones centrales y su distribución. In: Neuroanatomía Clínica. 6ª ed. Buenos Aires: Médica Panamericana; 2007. pp. 357-369

[55] Brennenstuhl H, Jung-Klawitter S, Assmann B, Opladen T. Inherited disorders of neurotransmitters: Classification and practical approaches for diagnosis and treatment. Neuropediatrics. 2019;**50**(1):2-14

[56] Cavanagh ME, Parnavelas JG. Neurotransmitter differentiation in cortical neurons. In: The Making of the Nervous System. London: Oxford Univ. Press; 1988. pp. 435-453

[57] Eroglu C, Barres BA. Regulation of synaptic connectivity by glia. Nature. 2010;**468**(7321):223-231

[58] Hassel B, Dingledine R. Glutamate and glutamate receptors. In: Basic Neurochemistry. Amsterdam, Netherlands: Academic Press; 2012. pp. 342-366

[59] Coghlan S, Horder J, Inkster B, Mendez MA, Murphy DG, Nutt DJ. GABA system dysfunction in autism and related disorders: From synapse to symptoms. Neuroscience and Biobehavioral Reviews. 2012;**36**:2044-2055

[60] Chao HT, Chen H, Samaco RC, Xue M, Chahrour M, Yoo J, et al. Dysfunction in GABA signalling mediates autism-like stereotypies and Rett syndrome phenotypes. Nature. 2010;**468**:263-269

[61] Cornell-Bell AH, Finkbeiner SM, Cooper MS, Smith SJ. Glutamate induces calcium waves in cultured astrocytes:

Long-range glial signaling. Science. 1990;**247**(4941):470-473

[62] Charles AC, Merrill JE, Dirksen ER, Sandersont MJ. Intercellular signaling in glial cells: Calcium waves and oscillations in response to mechanical stimulation and glutamate. Neuron. 1991;**6**(6):983-992

[63] Nedergaard M. Direct signaling from astrocytes to neurons in cultures of mammalian brain cells. Science. 1994;**263**(5154):1768-1771

[64] Smith SJ. Neural signalling: Neuromodulatory astrocytes. Current Biology. 1994;**4**(9):807-810

[65] Panatier A, Vallée J, Haber M, Murai KK, Lacaille JC, Robitaille R. Astrocytes are endogenous regulators of basal transmission at central synapses. Cell. 2011;**146**(5):785-798

[66] Gordon GR, Iremonger KJ, Kantevari S, Ellis-Davies GC, MacVicar BA, Bains JS. Astrocyte-mediated distributed plasticity at hypothalamic glutamate synapses. Neuron. 2009;**64**(3):391-403

[67] Rosenegger DG, Gordon GR. A slow or modulatory role of astrocytes in neurovascular coupling. Microcirculation. 2015;**22**(3):197-203

[68] Spanaki C, Kotzamani D, Petraki Z, Drakos E, Plaitakis A. Heterogeneous cellular distribution of glutamate dehydrogenase in brain and in non-neural tissues. Neurochemical Research. 2014;**39**:500-515

[69] Tasker JG, Oliet SH, Bains JS, Brown CH, Stern JE. Glial regulation of neuronal function: From synapse to systems physiology. Journal of Neuroendocrinology. 2012;**24**(4):566-576

[70] Morland C, Nordengen K. N-acetyl-aspartyl-glutamate in brain health and disease. International Journal of Molecular Sciences. 2022;**23**(3):1268

[71] Shave E, Pliss L, Lawrance ML, Fitz Gibbon T, Stastny F, Balcar VJ. Regional distribution and pharmacological characteristics of [3H] N-acetyl-aspartyl-glutamate (NAAG) binding sites in rat brain. Neurochemistry International. 2001;**38**(1):53-62

[72] Baslow MH. Evidence that the tri-cellular metabolism of N-acetylaspartate functions as the brain's "operating system": How NAA metabolism supports meaningful intercellular frequency-encoded communications. Amino Acids. 2010;**39**:1139-1145

[73] Baron-Cohen, S. La Gran Diferencia: Cómo son Realmente los Cerebros de Hombres y Mujeres 2005; Editorial AMAT: Barcelona, Spain; 2005

[74] Jiménez-Espinoza C, Rodríguez B, González M, Garrote M, González-Mora JL. Autism-Spectrum quotient (AQ): A preliminary study of its diagnostic validity in a clinical Spanish sample, more than a psychometric test? In: Proceedings of the International Meeting for Autism Research (IMFAR), Salt Lake City, UT, USA. ResearchGate Community, website and search engine. Berlín, Alemania. 13-16 May 2015

[75] Khachadourian V, Mahjani B, Sandin S, Kolevzon A, Buxbaum JD, Reichenberg A, et al. Comorbidities in autism spectrum disorder and their etiologies. Translational Psychiatry. 2023;**13**(1):71

[76] Govindaraju V, Young K, Maudsley AA. Proton NMR chemical shifts and coupling constants for brain metabolites. NMR in Biomedicine. 2000;**13**:129-153

[77] Provencher SW. Automatic quantitation of localized *in vivo*

1H spectra with LCModel. NMR in Biomedicine: An International Journal Devoted to the Development and Application of Magnetic Resonance *In Vivo*. 2001;**14**(4):260-264

[78] Cramér H. A contribution to the theory of statistical estimation. Scandinavian Actuarial Journal. 1946;**1946**:85-94

[79] De Graaf RA. *In Vivo* NMR Spectroscopy: Principles and Techniques. Hoboken, NJ, USA: John Wiley and Sons; 2013

[80] Edden RA, Pomper MG, Barker PB. *In vivo* differentiation of N-acetyl aspartyl glutamate from N-acetyl aspartate at 3 tesla. Magnetic Resonance in Medicine. 2007;**57**:977-982

[81] Savic I, Lekvall A, Greitz D, Helms G. MR spectroscopy shows reduced frontal lobe concentrations of N-acetyl aspartate in patients with juvenile myoclonic epilepsy. Epilepsia. 2000;**41**:290-296

[82] Haki C, Gümüştaş OG, Bora I, Gümüştaş AU, Parlak M. Proton magnetic resonance spectroscopy study of bilateral thalamus in juvenile myoclonic epilepsy. Seizure. 2007;**16**(4):287-295

[83] Lin K, Carrete H Jr, Lin J, Peruchi MM, De Araújo Filho GM, Guaranha MS, et al. Magnetic resonance spectroscopy reveals an epileptic network in juvenile myoclonic epilepsy. Epilepsia. 2009;**50**(5):1191-1200

[84] Helms G, Stawiarz L, KKP K, Link H. Regression analysis of metabolite concentrations estimated from localized proton MRspectra of active and chronic multiple sclerosis lesions. Magnetic Resonance in Medicine. 2000;**43**:102-110

[85] Brief EE, Vavasour IM, Laule C, Li DK, Mackay AL. Proton MRS of large multiple sclerosis lesions reveals subtle changes in metabolite T1 and area. NMR in Biomedicine. 2010;**23**(9):1033-1037

[86] Kirov II, Liu S, Tal A, Wu WE, Davitz MS, Babb JS, et al. Proton MR spectroscopy of lesion evolution in multiple sclerosis: Steady-state metabolism and its relationship to conventional imaging. Human Brain Mapping. 2017;**38**(8):4047-4063

[87] Chong VFH, Rumpel H, Aw Y-S, Ho G-L, Fan Y-F, Chua E-J. Temporal lobe necrosis following radiation therapy for nasopharyngeal carcinoma: 1H MR spectroscopic findings. International Journal of Radiation Oncology, Biology, Physics. 1999;**45**:699-705

[88] Chen WS, Li JJ, Zhang JH, Hong L, Xing ZB, Wang F, et al. Magnetic resonance spectroscopic imaging of brain injury after nasopharyngeal cancer radiation in early delayed reaction. Genetics and Molecular Research. 2014;**13**(3):6848-6854

[89] Rose SE, de Zubicaray GI, Wang D, Galloway GJ, Chalk JB, Eagle SC, et al. A 1H MRS study of probable Alzheimer's disease and normal aging: Implications for longitudinal monitoring of dementia progression. Magnetic resonance imaging. 1999;**17**:291-299

[90] Wang H, Tan L, Wang HF, Liu Y, Yin RH, Wang WY, et al. Magnetic resonance spectroscopy in Alzheimer's disease: Systematic review and meta-analysis. Journal of Alzheimer's Disease. 2015;**46**(4):1049-1070

[91] Pioro EP, Majors AW, Mitsumoto H, Nelson DR. Ng TC.1H-MRSevidence of neurodegeneration and excess glutamate+glutamine in ALS medulla. Neurology. 1999;**53**:71-79

[92] Targosz-Gajniak MG, Siuda JS, Wicher MM, Banasik TJ, Bujak MA, Augusciak-Duma AM, et al. Magnetic resonance spectroscopy as a predictor of conversion of mild cognitive impairment to dementia. Journal of the Neurological Sciences. 2013;**335**(1-2):58-63

[93] Zand DJ, Simon EM, Pulitzer SB, Wang DJ, Wang ZJ, Rorke LB, et al. *In vivo* pyruvate detected by MR spectroscopy in neonatal pyruvate dehydrogenase deficiency. American Journal of Neuroradiology. 2003;**24**(7):1471-1474

[94] Wilichowski E, Pouwels PJW, Frahm J, Hanefeld F. Quantitative proton magnetic resonance spectroscopy of cerebral metabolic disturbances in patients with MELAS. Neuropediatrics. 1999;**30**:256-263

[95] Wang R, Hu B, Sun C, Geng D, Lin J, Li Y. Metabolic abnormality in acute stroke-like lesion and its relationship with focal cerebral blood flow in patients with MELAS: Evidence from proton MR spectroscopy and arterial spin labeling. Mitochondrion. 2021;**1**(59):276-282

[96] Bernardino I, Dionísio A, Violante IR, Monteiro R, Castelo-Branco M. Motor cortex excitation/inhibition imbalance in young adults with autism spectrum disorder: A MRS-TMS approach. Frontiers in Psychiatry. 2022;**14**(13):860448

[97] Bejjani A, O'Neill J, Kim JA, Frew AJ, Yee VW, Ly R, et al. Elevated glutamatergic compounds in pregenual anterior cingulate in pediatric autism spectrum disorder demonstrated by 1H MRS and 1H MRSI. PLoS One. 2012;**7**(7):e38786

[98] Tebartz van Elst L, Maier S, Fangmeier T, Endres D, Mueller GT, Nickel K, et al. Disturbed cingulate glutamate metabolism in adults with high-functioning autism spectrum disorder: Evidence in support of the excitatory/inhibitory imbalance hypothesis. Molecular Psychiatry. 2014;**19**(12):1314-1325

[99] Foster TC. Calcium homeostasis and modulation of synaptic plasticity in the aged brain. Aging Cell. 2007;**6**(3):319-325

[100] Masuda F, Nakajima S, Miyazaki T, Yoshida K, Tsugawa S, Wada M, et al. Motor cortex excitability and inhibitory imbalance in autism spectrum disorder assessed with transcranial magnetic stimulation: A systematic review. Translational Psychiatry. 2019;**9**(1):110

[101] Watanabe T, Rees G. Anatomical imbalance between cortical networks in autism. Scientific Reports. 2016;**6**(1):31114

[102] Uddin LQ. Salience Network of the Human Brain. Amsterdam, Netherlands: Academic Press; 2016

[103] Schüz A, Miller R, editors. Cortical Areas: Unity and Diversity. Vol. 5. London, UK: CRC Press; 30 May 2002

Chapter 4

Glutamate Transporters in Health and Disease

Katelyn L. Reeb, Simran K. Gill, Rhea Temmermand and Andréia C.K. Fontana

Abstract

Glutamate transporters, or excitatory amino acid transporters (EAATs), are key proteins that regulate the excitatory tone in the central nervous system (CNS) by clearing synaptic glutamate, maintaining extracellular glutamate concentrations low enough to prevent receptor desensitization and/or glutamate-mediated excitotoxicity. Dysregulation of the function and/or expression of the EAATs is implicated in several diseases, including epilepsy, stroke, traumatic brain injury, drug abuse disorders, neurodegenerative disorders, and neuropathic pain, among others. In this chapter, we will discuss the regulatory mechanisms of EAATs in health and disease states. We will discuss post-translational modifications, trafficking deficits, reverse transport, and other regulatory processes. We will also discuss current approaches on potential therapeutic strategies targeting these transporters for many neuropsychiatric diseases.

Keywords: glutamate, glutamate transporters, EAAT, EAAT2, expression enhancers, GLT-1, ischemia, neuropathic pain, stroke, drug use disorder, allosteric modulation

1. Introduction

Glutamate transporters, or excitatory amino acid transporters (EAATs), play a crucial role in regulating excitatory activity in the central nervous system (CNS). Thus, studying their regulation is essential for understanding health and diseased states. In physiological states, glutamate is involved in memory, learning, and other processes, and EAATs exert a tight control of the synaptic concentration of glutamate, through clearance into glial and neuronal cells. In diseased states, glutamate transporter function and/or expression can be dysregulated, leading to devastating effects in the CNS. Under conditions of prolonged glutamate activation, cells become overexcited by glutamate and go through degeneration and, ultimately, death, in a process called excitotoxicity [1]. Glutamate-mediated excitotoxicity has been shown to be involved in numerous conditions, such as ischemic stroke, epilepsy, and traumatic brain injury. Further, dysregulated levels of glutamate transporters that result in abnormal synaptic glutamate concentration are observed in several pathologies, such as drug abuse disorders, neurodegenerative disorders, and neuropathic pain, among others. In this chapter, we will discuss the regulatory mechanisms of EAATs in physiological states and the implication of glutamate transporter dysregulation in neurological and neuropsychiatric disorders.

2. Glutamate transporters in health

In the mammalian CNS, glutamate serves as the main excitatory neurotransmitter and is a critical signal for neural communication and plasticity. Once released into the synaptic cleft, glutamate promotes specific signaling pathways in post-synaptic neurons by interacting with ionotropic and metabotropic glutamate receptors, which initiate downstream signaling. As extracellular glutamate cannot be enzymatically degraded, glutamate must be removed from the synaptic cleft through glutamate transporters [2]. Therefore, EAATs are imperative for proper neuronal functioning, as they clear synaptic glutamate and maintain excitatory balance.

2.1 Subtypes and localization in the nervous system

There are two main classes of glutamate transporters: EAATs, which are dependent on an electrochemical gradient of sodium (Na^+) ions, and the vesicular glutamate transporters (VGLUT-1-3) and cystine-glutamate antiporters (xCT), which are Na^+-independent (**Table 1**). EAATs and xCT are both found in cell membranes; however, xCT has much lower expression than the EAATs, whereas vGLUTs are found in the membrane of glutamate-containing synaptic vesicles. In this chapter, we will focus on EAATs. For a review of the xCT system, see [3]; for a review of vGLUTs, see [4].

EAATs are classified into five subtypes (rat/human homolog/gene): GLAST/EAAT1/SLC1A3, GLT-1/EAAT2/ SLC1A2, EAAC1/EAAT3/ SLC1A1, EAAT4/SLC1A6, and EAAT5/SLC1A7 [2]. EAAT1 and EAAT2 are mainly localized in astrocytes, whereas EAAT3-5 are neuronal [5]. The main transporters responsible for the uptake of synaptic glutamate are astrocytic EAAT1 and EAAT2; thus, they are key for preventing the accumulation of synaptic glutamate an avoid excitotoxicity [6]. EAAT1 is predominantly expressed in astrocytes within the cerebellar Purkinje cell layer [7]. EAAT2 is the predominant subtype of glutamate transporter in the CNS [8] and is expressed in astrocytes, select presynaptic neurons, and oligodendrocytes within the brain and spinal cord [9]. EAAT2 expression contributes to around 95% of total glutamate transport activity and represents approximately 1% of the total brain protein in the CNS [10], therefore, playing a key role in the maintenance of extracellular glutamate homeostasis. While both EAAT1 and EAAT2 are expressed within the same astrocytic plasma membrane, they are regulated differently; exogenous glutamate levels affect the cell-surface expression of EAAT1, but not EAAT2; EAAT2 is regulated by neuronal soluble factors, unlike EAAT1 [11]. Several splice variants of EAAT2 have been identified, with EAAT2b (or GLT-1b) being the most extensively studied. However, apparent functional differences between each of the variants are not readily apparent [12]. EAAT3 exhibits ubiquitous expression in the brain, playing a crucial role in regulating local glutamate concentrations, as it is predominantly located within post-synapsis, which allows for the buffering of nearby glutamate receptors, influencing excitatory neurotransmission and synaptic plasticity [13]. EAAT4, which is expressed in cerebellar neurons, is primarily responsible for maintaining

Glutamate transporter subtype-Human homolog	Glutamate transporter subtype-Rodent homolog	Gene	Cell type	Anatomic localization
EAAT1	GLAST	SLC1A3	Astrocytes, oligodendrocytes	Cerebellum, cortex, spinal cord Also, in testis and bone
EAAT2	GLT-1	SLC1A2	Mainly astroglia	Throughout brain and spinal cord Also, in liver
EAAT2b	GLT-1b	SLC1A2	Mainly astroglia, also expressed in neurons	Throughout brain and spinal cord Also in intestine, kidney, liver, and heart
EAAT3	EAAC1	SLC1A1	Neurons (dendrites and axon terminals)	Hippocampus, cerebellum, striatum
EAAT4	EAAT4	SLC1A6	Neurons (Purkinje cells)	Cerebellum, hippocampus, and basal ganglia Also, in placenta
EAAT5	EAAT5	SLC1A7	Neurons (photoreceptors and bipolar cells)	Retina Also, in liver
VGLUT1	VGLUT1	SLC17A7	Neurons	Cerebral cortex, hippocampus, and cerebellum
VGLUT2	VGLUT2	SLC17A6	Neurons	Thalamus and brainstem
VGLUT3	VGLUT3	SLC17A8	Neurons	Cerebral cortex, hippocampus, striatum, and raphe nuclei
xCT	xCT	SLC7A11	Neurons and glia	Hippocampus, cortex, hypothalamus, and dentate gyrus

Table 1.
Glutamate transporters: nomenclature (human/rodent/genes), cell type and anatomic localization.

low extracellular glutamate levels and preventing neurotoxicity in the cerebellum, together with glial EAAT1 [14]. EAAT5, a neuronal transporter mainly expressed in retina, plays a vital role in controlling glutamate release and mediating light responses in depolarizing bipolar cells in the retina [15].

See **Figure 1** for an overview of the localization of EAATs in the CNS.

2.2 Stoichiometry and structure of the EAATs

EAATs function through an electrogenic process that is dependent on the co-transport of three Na^+ (sodium) ions and one proton with glutamate and the counter-transport of one K^+ (potassium) ion out of the cell, in addition to an uncoupled Cl^- (chloride) current (**Figure 2A**) [16, 17]. This process is also known as an "induced fit mechanism," as Na^+ binding is required for glutamate binding, which also contributes to the high selectivity of EAATs for glutamate [18]. As EAATs are secondary

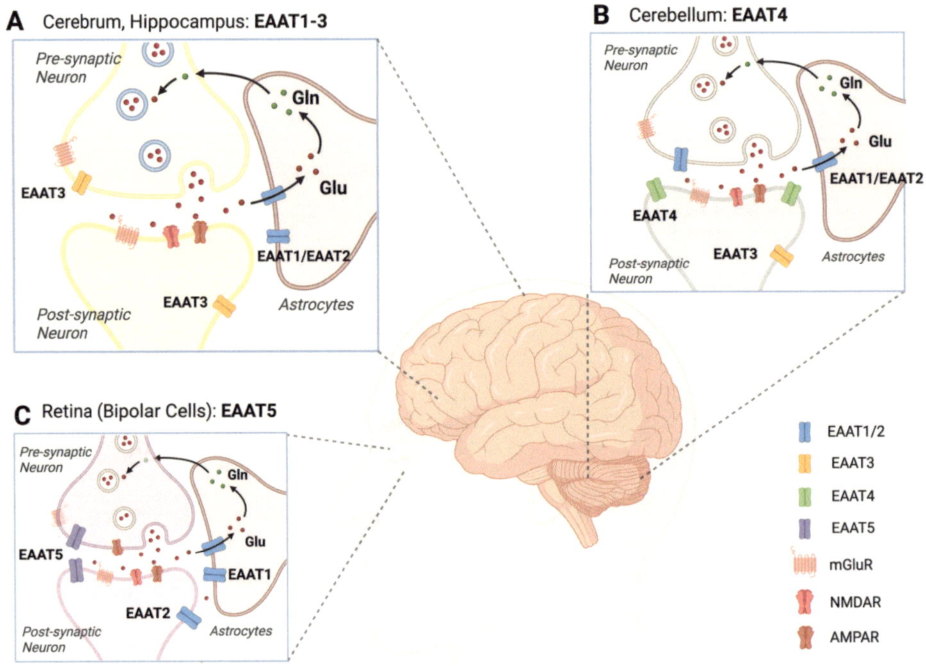

Figure 1.
Localization of neuronal and astrocytic excitatory amino acid transporters (EAATs) in the CNS. A. Overview of a glutamate tripartite synapse (pre- and post-synaptic neurons and astrocytes) showing the localization of astrocytic transporters EAAT1 and EAAT2 and neuronal transporter EAAT3, in the cerebrum and hippocampus. After glutamate (Glu, red dots) is released from the presynaptic terminal and stimulates postsynaptic glutamate receptors AMPA (α-amino-3-hydroxy-5-methyl-4-isoxazolepropionic) and NMDA (N-methyl-D-aspartate), and metabotropic glutamate receptors (mGluRs), it undergoes reuptake through EAATs present in astrocytes and neurons. In astrocytes, glutamate is converted into glutamine (Gln, green dots), which is shuttled back to neurons. In addition to glutamate, EAAT3 also transports the glutathione precursor cysteine (not shown) into neurons, which is required to produce glutathione. B. Overview of a glutamate tripartite synapse (pre- and post-synaptic neurons and astrocytes) showing the localization of astrocytic transporters EAAT1 and EAAT2 and neuronal transporters EAAT3 and EAAT4 in the cerebellum. Note that EAAT4 is only expressed in synapses in the cerebellum. C. Overview of a glutamate tripartite synapse (pre- and post-synaptic neurons and astrocytes) showing the localization of astrocytic transporter EAAT1 and EAAT2. Note that EAAT2, in the retina, is mainly expressed in neurons such as photoreceptors and bipolar cells, and neuronal transporter EAAT5 is only expressed in bipolar cells neurons in the retina. EAAT5 is restricted to. Created with BioRender.

active transporters, the ionic gradients of these substrates facilitate the glutamate transport cycle. EAATs rely indirectly on Na^+/K^+-ATPase (NKA) to generate these ion gradients [19].

EAATs are transmembrane integral proteins that traverse the cell membrane eight times (**Figure 2B**). EAATs consist of three protomers that can independently transport glutamate [16]. They have four key domains: a scaffold domain, or trimerization domain (comprised of transmembrane domains 1, 2, 4, 5), which remains stationary; a transporter domain (transmembrane domains 3, 6, 7, 8) that moves as a large rigid body along the scaffold domain in a twisting elevator-like motion to transport glutamate and its cosubstrates into the cell, and two hairpin domains (hairpin domains 1 and 2) that act as intracellular and extracellular gates [20]. These transporters follow an "alternating-access model" through this motion, which brings the transporter from an outward-facing conformation, where glutamate and cosubstrates bind, to an inward-facing conformation, where they are released (**Figure 2C**) [21]. While transporters

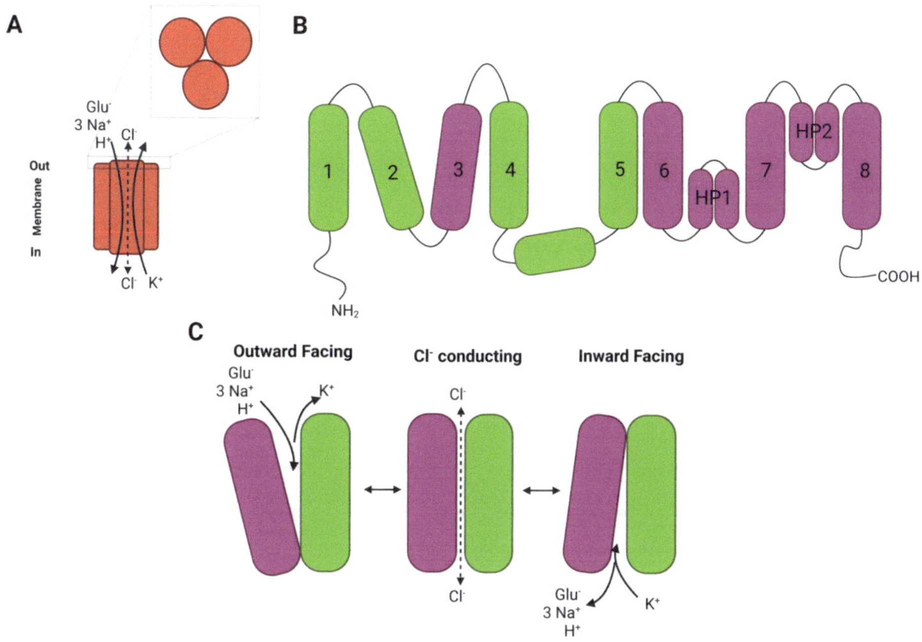

Figure 2.
Molecular properties of EAATs. A. Schematic displaying substrate stoichiometry associated with glutamate transport, displayed as trimer in the membrane. Glutamate (Glu) uptake is driven by co-transport of three Na^+ ions and one proton (H^+) and by counter-transport of one K^+ ion. EAATs also show an uncoupled Cl^- conductance (shown as dotted arrow). B. Transmembrane topology of glutamate transporters consisting of eight transmembrane domains and two hairpin loops (HP1 and HP2). Transmembrane domains are shown in dark blue, and scaffold domains in light blue. C. Glutamate transport cycle of a single protomer. Transport domain (magenta) of protomer moves along the scaffold domain (green) to go from an outward-facing conformation (far left) to an inward conformation (far right), passing through an intermediate conformation in which chloride conductance can occur. Created with BioRender.

and ion channels have historically been viewed as distinct proteins, EAATs also function as anion channels, which open during an intermediate state of the transport cycle [22]. This anion channel in EAATs is selective for chloride and is stoichiometrically uncoupled from glutamate transport [23]. Additionally, this chloride conductance may mediate neuronal excitability and ion homeostasis [24]. The malfunction of this chloride channel has also been linked to neurological diseases such as episodic ataxia [25]. Recent cryo-EM studies have reported the structures of EAAT1 [26], EAAT3 [27], and EAAT2 [28, 29] in several states in the presence of substrate glutamate or inhibitors. These studies are highly relevant as they revealed the structural basis of coupled substrate and ion binding.

2.3 Modulators of the activity of EAATs

In the last decades, compounds that modulate EAAT functions, directly or indirectly, have been identified and developed (some examples are outlined in **Table 2**).

Several compounds indirectly interact with EAATs, augmenting their catalytic activity, usually acting through multiple mechanisms, such as riluzole [30–43, 66]. Inhibitors of EAAT activity are grouped into competitive (bind to the same binding sites as glutamate) and non-competitive (bind somewhere else, i.e., to an allosteric

Compound	Mechanisms	References
Indirect activators		
Riluzole (2-amino 6-(trifluoromethoxy) benzothiazole)	• Increases activity and expression of EAAT2 • Blocks sodium channels	[30–43]
Positive allosteric modulators (PAMs)		
Parawixin1 (unknown chemical structure)	• Activates EAAT2 activity	[44]
GT949 (3-((4-Cyclohexylpiperazin-1-yl) (1-phenethyl-1H-tetrazol-5-yl) methyl)-6-methoxyquinolin-2(1H)-one and GT951 6-methoxy-3-((1-phenethyl-1H-tetrazol-5-yl) (4-(3-(trifluoromethyl) phenyl) piperazin-1-yl) methyl) quinolin-2(1H)-one)	• EAAT2 PAMs, activity, no effect on NMDA-mediated currents • *In vitro* neuroprotection in glutamate-mediated excitotoxicity models	[45, 46]
Parawixin10 (S)-N1-(3-(2-amino-5-guanidinopentanamido)propyl)-N4-(3-(2-(4-hydroxy-1H-indol-3-yl)acetamido) propyl)-N1,N1,N4,N4-tetramethylbutane-1,4-diaminium iodide)	• Increases glutamate uptake in rat brain synaptosomes. • PAM of EAAT1 and EAAT2 • Offers neuroprotection in *in vitro* stroke models and *in vivo* epilepsy models	[47–50]
[(*R*)-AS-1] [(R)- N-Benzyl-2-(2,5-dioxopyrrolidin-1-yl)propanamide)]	• Selective EAAT2 PAM • Offers *in vivo* protection from seizures	[51]
Competitive Inhibitors		
DL-TBOA and analogs (DL-threo-beta-benzyloxy aspartate)	• Non-transportable blocker of all subtypes of EAATs	[52–60]
TFB-TBOA *[*(3S)-3-[[3-[[4-(Trifluoromethyl) benzoyl] amino] phenyl] methoxy]-L-aspartic acid]	• Selective inhibitor of EAAT1 and EAAT2	[61–64]
Non-competitive inhibitors		
Several putative negative allosteric modulators	• Selective and non-selective inhibition of EAAT1, EAAT2, and/or EAAT3	[65]

The table includes indirect activators (compounds that interact indirectly with EAATs augmenting their catalytic activity, usually acting through multiple mechanisms), positive allosteric modulators (PAMs, compounds that interact directly with EAATs at an allosteric site and putatively increase their activity), competitive inhibitors (compounds that bind to the same binding sites as glutamate, competing with glutamate for binding to the transporter protein; some of these inhibitors are substrates themselves, some are exchanged with internal glutamate and induce glutamate release), and non-competitive inhibitors (or negative allosteric modulators, NAMs, that act by binding EAATs at an allosteric site, often leading to a conformational change that impacts transporter dynamics). In addition, we provide some of their known mechanisms and include further references.

Table 2.
Examples of modulators of excitatory amino acid (EAAT) activity.

site). Some of these inhibitors are substrates themselves, and some are exchanged with internal glutamate, thereby inducing glutamate release [52].

An emerging approach to drug design focuses on allosteric modulators, which bind to allosteric sites and alter the conformation of the orthosteric binding site, affecting transport by either enhancing (positive allosteric modulation, PAM) or inhibiting (negative allosteric modulation, NAM) binding affinity and transport.

Allosteric modulation may offer advantages such as targeted drug therapy and increased specificity, thus offering promising prospects for drug discovery and the development of novel therapeutics [67]. Recently, allosteric sites have been described in EAATs [45, 46]. The development of selective EAAT PAMs and NAMs may be useful tools to decipher how drugs can affect the transport cycle and to investigate the intrinsic properties and functions of the EAATs [68].

Further research on allosteric modulators of EAATs is necessary to address several outstanding questions. These include determining the precise location and physiological significance of the allosteric binding sites, investigating whether these compounds can stabilize specific conformations of the transporter, understanding how different conformations of EAATs transmit signals into the cell, and exploring the possibility of allosterically modulating transporter-mediated efflux. Ultimately, this knowledge could be invaluable for advancing our understanding of EAAT modulation and for informing the drug development process [69].

2.4 Modulators of the expression of EAATs

The expression of EAATs is altered in certain disease states, leading to changes in neuronal excitation. This regulation can occur through transcriptional and translational processes [70]. However, the exact mechanisms underlying EAATs expression regulation are not well understood; hence, synthetic modulators of expression could serve as valuable tools for investigating the functions and regulation of EAATs in both physiological and disease contexts. There are exogenous drugs, endogenous molecules, and proteins that increase EAATs expression (transcriptional and level, i.e., increase gene transcription, and translational, i.e., increase the protein expression) and inhibitors of EAAT expression. Additional research is needed to evaluate whether a compound that enhances GLT-1 expression and has good brain penetrance, favorable pharmacokinetic properties, and low risk of side effects and toxicity can be developed into a therapeutic drug [71]. Some commonly studied EAAT expression modulators are outlined in **Table 3**.

2.5 Trafficking and post-translational modifications of EAATs

The expression and function of EAATs are regulated at the genetic, epigenetic, transcriptional, post-transcriptional, and translational levels [132]. Dysregulation of these processes can lead to severe outcomes such as high levels of extracellular glutamate and excitotoxicity [6]. The activity of transporters can be regulated by many means, such as ubiquitination, phosphorylation glycosylation, and sulfhydryl oxidation, among others [133–135].

Post-translational modification of GLT-1 by ubiquitin conjugation to lysine residues has been found to mediate the transporters constitutive internalization and degradation. This regulated clathrin-mediated endocytosis in basal conditions determines the availability of transporter on the cell surface and therefore relates directly to activity levels and rate of glutamate transport [123, 136]. Additionally, the palmitoylation of GLT-1 has been shown to drive glutamate uptake kinetics. Palmitoylation involves the covalent attachment of palmitic acid to one of more cysteine residues of the target protein. Studies suggest that palmitoylation of GLT-1 is important for glutamate uptake capacity, as a reduction in palmitoylated GLT-1 leads to impairments in glutamate clearance [137]. The sumoylation of GLT-1 in physiological signaling has also been identified, which involves the attachment of a SUMO

Compound	Mechanism	References
Expression enhancers		
Ceftriaxone ((6R,7R)-7-{[(2Z)-2-(2-amino-1,3-thiazol-4-yl)- > 2-(methoxyimino) acetyl]amino} MI-3-{[(2-methyl-5,6-dioxo-1,2,5,6-tetrahydro-1,2,4-triazin-3-yl)thio]methyl}-8-oxo-5-thia-1-azabicyclo[4.2.0]oct-2-ene-2-carboxylic acid)	• β-Lactam antibiotic • Selective enhancer of EAAT2 expression, through transcriptional activation via mechanisms involving PI3K/Akt/NF-κB	[72–100]
Clavulanic acid ((2R,5R, Z)-3-(2-hydroxyethylidene)-7-oxo-4-oxa-1-aza-bicyclo [3.2.0] heptane-2-carboxylic acid)	• Structural analog β-lactam but lacks antibiotic effects • Increases EAAT2 expression (has better oral availability and blood-brain barrier penetration than ceftriaxone)	[77, 79, 101–106]
LDN/OSU-0212320 (Thiopyridazine and pyridazine derivatives)	• Increases EAAT2 expression through translational activation	[107–112]
Amitriptyline (3-(10,11-dihydro-5H-dibenzo [a, d] cycloheptene-5-ylidene)-N, N-dimethylpropan-1-amine)	• Tricyclic antidepressant • Induces EAAT2 expression and ameliorates neuropathic pain	[113, 114]
N-acetylcysteine ((2R)-2-acetamido-3-sulfanylpropanoic acid))	• Increases EAAT2 expression- • Reduces drug-seeking/taking behavior for cocaine, nicotine, and ethanol	[115–121]
Minocycline ((2E,4S,4aR,5aS,12aR)-2-(Amino-hydroxy -methylidene)-4,7-bis(dimethylamino)-10,11,12a-trihydroxy-4a,5,5a,6-tetrahydro-4H-tetracene-1,3,12-trione)	• Broad-spectrum tetracycline antibiotic • Ameliorates downregulation of GLT-1 expression in neuropathy model	[122]
Expression inhibitors		
PMA (phorbol 12-myristate 13-acetate)	• Activator of PKC • Decreases the activity and expression of GLT-1 through clathrin-mediated endocytosis • (Also has actions on EAAT3)	[123–128]
Synthetic cathinone MDPV (3,4-methylenedioxypyrovalerone methylenedioxy pyrovalerone)	• Downregulates GLT-1 expression, and norepinephrine-dopamine reuptake	[129]
Amphetamine (1-phenylpropan-2-amine)	• Potent CNS stimulant • Downregulates EAAT3 expression • Enters dopamine neurons via DAT and triggers endocytosis of EAAT3, in a process involving dynamin- and Rho-mediated mechanisms	[130, 131]

The table includes examples of drugs that enhance EAATs expression (at the transcriptional and translational level), and examples of drugs that inhibit EAATs expression, along with some of their known mechanisms and further references.

Table 3.
Examples of modulators of Excitatory Amino Acid Transporters (EAAT) expression.

protein to a lysine residue on the target protein and was found to regulate GLT-1 subcellular localization [138]. Notably, several groups have reported aberrations in the constitutive trafficking, expression, and activity levels of glutamate transporters due to alterations in post-translational modifications in many disease states, which will be further discussed in Section 3.

3. Glutamate transporters in disease

Dysregulation of EAATs plays a significant role in many neuropsychiatric diseases/disorders. Below, we briefly discuss two mechanisms of EAAT dysregulation involved in several disorders: glutamate efflux *via* transporter reversal and downregulation of the expression of glutamate transporters. We also briefly describe studies of knockout of EAAT that were pivotal for our understanding of the role of glutamate transporters in health and disease.

3.1 Glutamate transporter reversal

Under physiological conditions, the direction of glutamate transport is inward; however, in pathological conditions, the function of Na^+/K^+-ATPase (NKA) becomes dysfunctional, with subsequent disruption of Na^+/K^+ electrochemical gradient needed for glutamate translocation, resulting in increases in extracellular K^+ and decreases in Na^+ decreases, which leads to glutamate transport in the outward direction [139]. In support of this, massive increases in extracellular K^+ and indiscriminate release of glutamate have been reported following concussive and lateral fluid percussion brain injuries [140], ischemia [141], and oxidative stress in a SOD1 mutation amyotrophic lateral sclerosis (ALS) model [142, 143].

It remains to be clarified whether EAAT functional activators or expression enhancers will facilitate glutamate clearance under excitotoxic conditions or will intensify reverse transport. However, previous preclinical studies suggest neuroprotective properties of these compound classes against ischemia, which encourages future drug development using this strategy. Nevertheless, as glutamatergic signaling plays crucial roles in brain development, cell survival, and synaptogenesis, these pharmacological strategies encounter similar challenges to other drugs targeting glutamate-mediated mechanisms, such as the potential for significant adverse effects [71, 144].

3.2 Glutamate transporter downregulation

Reduced expression and function of EAATs has been reported in numerous neurological disorders. Although the exact mechanism of downregulation has yet to be fully established, it results in impairment of the overall function of glutamate transporters, which plays an important role in the etiology of neurological diseases (see below).

For an overview of the role of EAATs at glutamatergic synapses at physiological (A) and pathological (B) states, see **Figure 3**.

3.3 Studies with knockout of EAATs

Studies with knockout of glutamate transporters reveal a major role for EAATs in clearance of glutamate, excitotoxicity, and associated neurotransmission. A key study by Tanaka's group in the 1990s demonstrated that EAAT2 gene knockout resulted in lethal

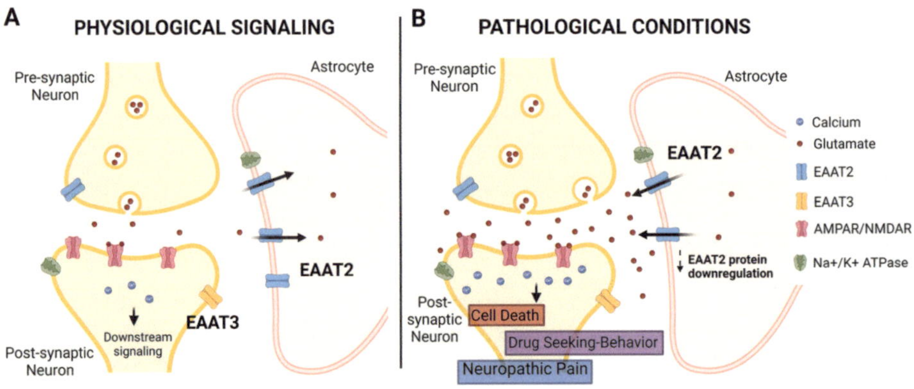

Figure 3.
Tripartite glutamatergic synapse in physiological and pathological conditions. Schematic representing glutamatergic transmission in the context of physiological (A) and pathological (B) states that are associated with glutamate-induced excitotoxicity and EAAT2 protein dysregulation. A. In B. Hyper-glutamatergic signaling results in excess glutamate (red dots) release, overactivation of ionotropic glutamate receptors AMPA and NMDA, and aberrant calcium (blue dots) influx leading to the activation of various cell death pathways. In many disease states, glutamatergic dysfunction can lead to transporter reversal (shown by the arrow pointing to glutamate efflux from the astrocytes to the extracellular environment) and downregulation (shown as lower EAAT2 expression than in A), further exacerbating excitotoxic outcomes, such as in ischemic stroke. Na+/K+ ATPase (NKA) dysfunction also contributes to the dysregulation of EAAT activity. Downregulation of EAAT2 expression is also observed in pathologies such as in drugs of abuse disorders (depicted in the figure as drug-seeking behavior) and neuropathic pain. Created with BioRender.

spontaneous seizures and increased susceptibility to acute cortical injury in mice [145]. Later studies confirmed severe disturbances in mice lacking GLT-1 and GLAST [146], including elevated extracellular glutamate levels, exacerbated hippocampal neuronal damage after brain injury [147], impairment of several essential aspects of neuronal development [148], neurodegeneration and progressive paralysis [149]. Mice lacking EAAT1 have decreased cerebellar function, reduced motor coordination, hearing loss, and disturbed retinal function. Antisense knockdown of GLAST compromises retinal function [150], and constitutive deletion of GLAST results in markedly reduced alcohol consumption and preference [151]. Mice lacking EAAT3 develop dicarboxylic aminoaciduria (Kegg's disease), exhibit reduced spontaneous locomotor activity, and may age prematurely [152]. Additionally, they experience depletion of glutathione and neuronal cell loss [153], suggesting that EAAT3 plays a critical role in providing cysteine for glutathione synthesis [154]. Humans lacking EAAT3 develop dicarboxylic aminoaciduria, a rare metabolic disorder that causes the body to excrete too much aspartate and glutamate in urine, and human EAAT3 polymorphisms have been reported to be associated with obsessive-compulsive disorders [155]. In EAAT4 knockout mice, Purkinje cells are more likely to die [156], and in a double knockout of EAAT1 and EAAT4, both highly expressed in the cerebellum, a differential effect was observed in the spontaneous firing pattern and survival of Purkinje cells [14], demonstrating the essential role of these transporters in the cerebellum. Finally, EAAT5 was shown to shape the retinal light responses, in an EAAT5 knockout model [157].

3.4 Stroke

Stroke is the third leading cause of death in the United States, accounting for 700,000 fatalities each year [158]. Following an ischemic event, inadequate blood flow to the brain prevents the delivery of oxygen and glucose. The deprivation of these substrates to neurons causes cell death and lasting brain damage [159]. Following a focal ischemic event, the resulting damage manifests into two distinct regions that are classified as the infarction core and the penumbra. The core is the region of the brain in which the primary occlusion occurs, which undergoes rapid and irreversible cellular death within minutes of ischemic onset, usually due to necrosis [160]. The penumbra is classified as the region that surrounds the core, which receives reduced blood supply but remains partially metabolically active and therefore contains salvageable tissue. However, this region is at risk of cell death if blood flow is not quickly restored [159], making the penumbra the primary area of interest for new targeted therapies.

Glutamatergic dysfunction is a key factor contributing to neuronal cell death following ischemic stroke [161, 162]. The lack of oxygen due to cessation of blood flow results in depleted ATP stores, thereby disrupting the ionic gradients responsible for regulating neuronal firing, resulting in increased action potentials and aberrant glutamatergic signaling. Excessive release of glutamate during ischemia leads to overactivation of postsynaptic ionotropic glutamate receptors. Released glutamate may also diffuse out of the synaptic cleft, causing activation of distant (extrasynaptic) receptors and subsequent elevated calcium influx into the cytosol. This affects calcium-sensitive organelles such as the mitochondria and endoplasmic reticulum [163] and causes the release of calcineurin and calpains, mediators of cell death [164]. Mitochondrial dysfunction and oxidative stress also play key parts in the excitotoxic phenotype [165]. Thus, minimizing glutamate-induced excitotoxicity by regulating the aberrant signaling cascade following stroke can be therapeutically beneficial in improving post-stroke outcomes.

As EAATs are responsible for removing glutamate from the synaptic space to help end neurotransmission, these proteins play a key role in mitigating excitotoxic outcomes. Recent research has focused on better understanding the regulation of EAATs during or after an ischemic event as well as on strategies to modulate their expression and/or activity to bolster glutamate clearance and promote cell recovery. Many groups have identified temporal and spatial alterations in glutamate transporter expression over the course of ischemic injury [166]. Additionally, the activity and function of glutamate transporters can be significantly affected by the severity of ischemic insult, with severe insults even causing a reversal in glutamate transport due to disruptions in the ionic gradients that drive these transporters [167]. Membrane translocation of glutamate transporters after ischemia has also been suggested, with elevations in glutamate release causing rapid changes in the diffusion and clustering of EAAT2 along the plasma membrane [168]. Taken together, the regulatory movement and response of glutamate transporters to ischemic insult is complex and multifaceted.

An extensively researched pathway in addressing ischemic injury involves the modulation of glutamate transporter expression. Pharmacological preconditioning with several β-lactam antibiotics, most notably ceftriaxone, an EAAT2 expression enhancer, has shown promising results as a treatment option in several neurological disorders including ischemic stroke. Previous work has found that ceftriaxone, when administered 48 hours before OGD, reduced neuronal death by 20–50%, thereby providing neuroprotection [72]. In this model, daily administration of ceftriaxone 5 days prior to middle cerebral artery occlusion (MCAO) provided neuroprotection through a reduction in infarct volume as well as neuroinflammatory and apoptotic factors through EAAT2 upregulation [73]. Additionally, a study found that daily administration of ceftriaxone as well as N-acetylcysteine 5 days prior to focal cerebral ischemia also significantly increased EAAT2 expression levels in addition to a reduction of infarct volume [115]. Other compounds that protect neurons from glutamate-induced excitotoxic death, such as LDN-OSU0212320, decrease infarct volume in mice when administered 24 hours prior to photothrombotic ischemia; however, only in male mice, suggesting that this treatment may not be effective in the female population and further emphasizing the importance of sex differences in targeted treatments [107, 108]. A significant drawback associated with β-lactam antibiotics in enhancing EAAT2 expression is the extended time required for drug onset (≥24 hours) [169]. Therefore, in the context of clinical ischemic injury, more fast-acting compounds need to be developed. EAAT PAMs offer a different approach to restoring glutamate clearance through the enhancement of glutamate uptake; however, this hypothesis remains to be tested in animal models of stroke.

3.5 Traumatic brain injury

Studies on traumatic brain injury (TBI) in both humans and animals have shown an acute increase in tissue glutamate concentrations that persist at elevated levels for up to 5 days in humans. This suggests a delay or insufficient glutamate clearance by glutamate transporters following TBI [71, 170]. Many studies have established that the subsequent glutamate-mediated excitotoxicity plays a significant role in acute post-injury neurodegenerative events [171]. In addition, decreased GLT-1 expression was shown in several TBI preclinical studies [147], which is consistent with the decreased EAAT2 activity observed in TBI patients [171]. Furthermore, antisense knockdown of GLT-1 in rat aggravates neuronal damage following TBI [172].

TBI is a complex pathology of many etiologies, which varies depending on the severity of the injury and the location of the affected brain tissue. In cases of concussion, where brain injury is typically reversible and symptoms resolve over time [173], the opportunity to reduce acute glutamate excitotoxicity by targeting GLT-1 offers potential for neuroprotection. However, for other types of TBI, additional pharmacological approaches may be necessary to address the diverse pathophysiological mechanisms involved [174].

3.6 Epilepsy

Epilepsy is a group of disorders characterized by recurrent spontaneous seizures that appear to stem from intricate processes involving various neurotransmitter systems, including glutamate [175, 176]. This leads to an imbalance between neuronal excitatory and inhibitory activities, ultimately culminating in epileptogenesis [177]. Numerous drugs are available as anti-seizure medications; however, none of the current treatments are considered disease-modifying, as they only suppress seizures without addressing the development and progression of epilepsy.

As previously mentioned, a key preclinical study revealed that mice lacking GLT-1 are prone to exhibit seizures [145]. Additionally, conditional deletion of GLT-1 revealed that GLT-1 protects against fatal epilepsy [178]. Loss of GLAST or GLT-1 led to elevated extracellular glutamate levels, neurodegeneration, and progressive paralysis, and loss of EAAC1 caused mild neurotoxicity and resulted in epilepsy [149]. In patients with medial temporal lobe epilepsy (mTLE), increased extracellular glutamate levels were observed [179] as well as decreased levels of EAAT1, EAAT2, and EAAT3 [180], reviewed in Ref. [176]. Decreased levels of GLT-1 were also observed in animal models of epilepsy such as pilocarpine-induced [181], albumin-induced [182], tuberous sclerosis-induced [183], $FeCl_3$-induced models [184], and chest compression-induced audiogenic model [185].

However, some studies did not observe changes in EAAT2 levels in patients [186] and in animal models including kindling [187], anticonvulsant ketogenic diet [188], and spontaneously epileptic rats [189], suggesting that EAAT2 may be implicated in the etiology of only some types of epilepsy. Another concept suggests that a deficiency in glutamine synthetase in astrocytes may be the molecular mechanism underlying extracellular glutamate accumulation and seizure generation [190].

Nonetheless, the upregulation of EAAT2 *via* transcriptional and translational regulation has demonstrated success *in vivo* by reducing spontaneous recurrent seizures and providing neuroprotection [191].

Parawixin10, a compound isolated from *Parawixia bistriata* spider venom, is a non-selective PAM of EAAT1 and EAAT2, with *in vitro* neuroprotective properties [47] and *in vivo* neuroprotection in epilepsy models of intrahippocampal injection of NMDA [48], kainic acid and pentylenetetrazol (PTZ) [49], and pilocarpine [50]. These studies served as *proof of concept* that EAAT1-2 PAMs may offer neuroprotection and anticonvulsant properties. More recently, the selective EAAT2 PAM [(*R*)-AS-1] revealed favorable anticonvulsant and safety profiles, and significant protection in mice against seizures in acute and chronic animal models of seizures [51]. These novel compounds may have disease-modifying potential in acquired epilepsy, which will require future experimental testing.

Several studies demonstrated mutations in EAAT1 are implicated in episodic ataxia 6 (EA6), a chronic condition characterized by epilepsy, nystagmus, and tinnitus. These mutations result in impaired glutamate uptake and alterations in anion conductance; however, how exactly these mutations affect EAAT1 expression, subcellular localization, function, and the complex neurological phenotype of EA6 remains to be understood [25].

Collectively, these studies suggest that astrocytic glutamate uptake plays a critical role in protecting neurons from hyperexcitability. However, discrepancies in some findings indicate that the exact mechanisms remain elusive. Nevertheless, the idea that modulating astrocytic EAATs represents a potential therapeutic approach to provide neuroprotection, to prevent spontaneous recurrent seizures, and to halt epileptogenesis [192].

3.7 Pain

Pain, an aversive sensory experience arising from actual or perceived tissue damage, constitutes a physiologic response to noxious stimuli or disease, serving as a protective mechanism to prompt seeking care or preventing further harm [193]. Pain perception involves complex interactions among cellular and molecular components, including neurons, glia, glutamate receptors, and transporters that utilize glutamate, the primary transmitter released by sensory afferents in the nervous system [194–196]. However, when pain extends beyond the acute injury phase, persisting for more than 3 months, it transitions into a chronic disease. Chronic pain, a prevalent motive for medical intervention, correlates with heightened risks of poor mental health, opioid dependency, and diminished quality of life.

During chronic pain development, excess glutamate released in the peripheral and central nervous system contributes to elevated extracellular glutamate levels, which overactivates glutamate receptors and exacerbates pain symptoms. Prolonged overactivation leads to neuroplasticity in pain pathways, amplifying pain signals, a phenomenon known as central sensitization [197]. Glutamate transporters, particularly EAAT2, counteract this process by removing extracellular glutamate and reducing pain signaling [196, 198]. In the pain pathway, EAAT2 is expressed in the anterior cingulate cortex, somatosensory cortex, hippocampus, and dorsal horn of the spinal cord [199].

After injury occurs, the expression of EAATs changes, potentially contributing to chronic pain conditions. Numerous pain models have been used to study EAATs during neuropathic pain development but with varying results. For example, in nerve-injury models of pain, studies found an initial increase in EAAT2 3–7 days after surgery, followed by a steep downregulation below baseline [200]. Other studies did not observe this initial upregulation in EAAT1 or EAAT2 early after injury and instead observed an upregulation of EAAT3 and a downregulation of EAAT1 and EAAT2 [101]. Because of these inconsistencies, the relationship between neuropathic pain development and EAAT expression remains unclear.

Various mechanisms are being explored for chronic pain therapy, and targeting the glutamatergic system to reduce pain transmission shows promising potential [196, 201]. Although glutamate receptor antagonism provides anti-nociception, it may be associated with severe side effects, including sedation, hallucinations, and cardiac instability, limiting its use in outpatient settings [202]. A potential novel therapeutic approach involves the modulation of astrocytic EAATs, located on cells that surround glutamatergic neurons, aiming to restore homeostasis by lowering the concentration of extracellular glutamate. In this sense, downregulation or inhibition of EAATs has been reported to increase pain [203], whereas increased EAAT2 expression can mitigate pain [204–206]. For example, overexpression of GLT-1 in the spinal cord attenuated the induction of inflammatory and neuropathic pain, suggesting this could be a strategy for pain [207]. Furthermore, positive allosteric modulation of EAATs can enhance their efficiency in various neurological diseases, offering neuroprotection, and is a potential target for chronic pain.

In preclinical pain models, certain drug classes have been shown to have anti-nociceptive properties by modulating EAATs through the enhancement of EAAT expression and removal of excessive glutamate [196, 203, 208]. Some of these drugs include β-lactam antibiotics (such as ceftriaxone), β-lactamase inhibitors (such as clavulanic acid), tetracycline antibiotics (such as minocycline), anticonvulsants (including VPA and riluzole), and tricyclic antidepressants (such as amitriptyline) [196]. Ceftriaxone has undergone extensive research as a potential therapy for modulating EAAT2 expression. Studies in the chronic constriction injury (CCI) pain model demonstrated that ceftriaxone upregulated GLT-1 expression and glutamate uptake in the spinal dorsal horn and resulted in anti-nociceptive effects [74, 75]. Furthermore, its impact extended to a model of multiple sclerosis, where ceftriaxone not only reversed tactile allodynia but also halted the progression of motor weakness and paralysis. Notably, in both models, ceftriaxone reversed the reduction in EAAT2 expression and astrocyte activation in the lumbar spinal cord, suggesting its potential to suppress glial activation and alleviate pain [75].

Concerns about the antibiotic activity of ceftriaxone led to the investigation of clavulanic acid, which is devoid of antibiotic properties. In the CCI model, both clavulanic acid and ceftriaxone demonstrated anti-nociception, increased EAAT2 expression in the rat spinal cord, and reversed EAAT2 downregulation at day 14 post-surgery [209]. Clavulanic acid may be a candidate for relieving pain in diabetic peripheral neuropathy, and its benefits could be attributed to increased EAAT2 expression [101].

Another approach to modulate EAAT2 that could be beneficial for various pain conditions is through positive allosteric modulation (PAM), which involves the enhancement of extracellular glutamate uptake. Several preclinical pain studies demonstrated a downregulation of EAAT2, thus enhancing the activity of the remaining transporters *via* PAM represents a promising new avenue for future drug development [196, 210]. Selective EAAT2 PAMs will restore glutamate homeostasis by enhancing the uptake of excessive glutamate, rather than blocking glutamatergic transmission; thus, this approach is expected to be safer and devoid of the dissociative effects observed with NMDA receptor antagonists [196]. Additionally, EAAT2 PAM compounds differ significantly from transcriptional or translational upregulation of EAAT2 expression, such as ceftriaxone, which display varying efficacies across individuals, raising concerns about safety, efficacy, and adverse effects. EAAT2 PAMs work directly on the transporter, rapidly increasing glutamate uptake efficiency, resulting in a quicker onset compared to drugs that modulate expression. They are highly selective, providing a more robust and safe clinical profile compared to epigenetic-modifying expression enhancers that are often associated with adverse side effects [196, 211]; however, further studies are needed to confirm these expectations.

3.8 Substance use disorders

The maintenance of low extracellular glutamate levels in the CNS is important for proper cognitive functions such as learning and memory [212]. Both learning and memory are involved in the cycle of addiction, as is evident by relapses [213]. Substance use disorder is characterized by compulsion to use a substance, inability to limit intake of that substance, and the appearance of negative affect following the use of the drug. Regions such as the prefrontal cortex, amygdala, and hippocampus, which are involved in learning and memory, have projections connecting them to key regions involved in addiction, such as the ventral tegmental area and nucleus accumbens [214]. Drug use activates glutamatergic neurotransmission in the mesocorticolimbic system [215]. Following repeated use, drug-specific changes occur in these brain regions that drive the susceptibility to relapse and chronic drug use [216]. Furthermore, in abuse models, dysregulation of glutamate levels is observed in key brain regions associated with addiction, such as the prefrontal cortex, hippocampus, and nucleus accumbens [217]. All drugs of abuse disrupt glutamate homeostasis during use, increasing synaptic glutamate release. Numerous studies have demonstrated the importance of glutamatergic signaling in the nucleus accumbens on drug-seeking [218]. The importance of changes in glutamatergic tone that occur in addiction is further evident as pharmacologically restoring glutamate levels reduces drug-seeking behavior [219].

Targeting EAAT2 specifically has displayed promising results in the context of addiction. The use of drugs such as cocaine, cannabinoids, amphetamine, ethanol, nicotine, and opiates results in significant changes in EAAT2 levels [216]. Preclinical studies have shown that ceftriaxone inhibits cue- and drug-induced reinstatement seeking for cocaine [220], heroin [221], methamphetamine [222], and nicotine [223]. Additionally, administration of ceftriaxone attenuates the development of cocaine-induced conditioned place and prevents the decrease in EAAT2 expression in the nucleus accumbens [224]. Ceftriaxone also reduces alcohol intake [76]. Clavulanic acid reduces the reinforcing efficacy of cocaine and reduces cocaine-conditioned place preference [77]. Additionally, clavulanic acid reduced morphine-conditioned place preference, morphine-induced hypothermia, and locomotor sensitization [102].

Riluzole prevents cocaine reinstatement while restoring the expression of EAAT2 in the nucleus accumbens [225]. However, clinical trials found that riluzole was not effective for cocaine use disorder, when taken during the period of cocaine dependency [226]. Interestingly, riluzole has shown some promising effects in clinical trials for methamphetamine dependence, as it decreased symptoms, such as craving, withdrawal, and depression, experienced by men in an outpatient setting [227]. This study was supported by previous findings that riluzole reduces methamphetamine-induced locomotor sensitization [228]. Additionally, riluzole affects morphine- and amphetamine-conditioned place preference [229]. Riluzole also reduced ethanol self-administration in mice [230]. N-acetylcysteine (NAC), an antioxidant cystine pro-drug, is an over-the-counter supplement that suppresses NF-κB [116], a transcriptional regulator of EAAT2 [117]. While NAC has low oral availability, NAC has been shown to restore EAAT2 expression and to reduce drug-seeking/taking behavior for cocaine [118], nicotine [119], and ethanol [120].

Another promising approach for targeting EAAT2 in the context of addiction is by increasing the efficiency of the transport through PAMs. EAAT2 PAMs offer the unique advantage of having a quick onset, which may be of critical importance during craving.

3.9 Neurodegenerative disorders

Alzheimer's disease (AD) is a progressive age-related neurodegenerative disorder characterized by abnormal deposition of fibrillar amyloid β (Aβ) protein, intracellular neurofibrillary tangles, oxidative damage, and tau protein hyperphosphorylation that contributes to neuronal dysfunction [231–233]. The aberrant glutamate stimulation that results in synaptic dysfunction has been proposed as one of several mechanisms of synaptic damage in AD. This is supported by studies reporting reduced GLT-1 expression and function in AD [234, 235] and post-mortem analysis of human brain tissue from patients with AD (as well as other neurodegenerative disorders), suggesting that EAAT2 loss or dysfunction could be an early trigger evolving into chronic reactive astrogliosis, oxidative stress, and neuronal death [236]. Also, a study demonstrated that Aβ1–42 prompts rapid GLT-1 mislocalization and internalization in astrocytes, reducing the rate of glutamate clearance [237]. Another study found that GLT-1 loss led to a compensatory increase in insulin-degrading enzyme activity in the liver, implicating partial GLT-1 loss in insulin/Akt signaling abnormalities observed in AD [238]. Further, a study suggested that decreased expression of glutamine synthetase but no changes in GLT-1 expression in a model of AD [239]. Thus, it is not yet entirely clear whether GLT-1/EAAT2 dysfunction plays a pathogenic role in AD and whether targeting this transporter may be developed as a neuroprotective strategy for the pathogenesis of AD.

Currently, available treatments for AD include acetylcholinesterase inhibitors [240], NMDA receptor antagonist memantine [241], and monoclonal antibody therapies that target the removal of β-amyloid from the brain such as lecanemab [242]. However, these treatments offer only symptomatic relief and primarily target late-stage aspects of the disease. Additionally, the efficacy of monoclonal antibodies has not been proven. Therefore, a definite treatment for this disease is yet to be identified.

Amyotrophic lateral sclerosis (ALS): ALS is a debilitating disease characterized by progressive loss of voluntary motor neurons, leading to muscle atrophy, weight loss, and respiratory failure [243]. The pathogenesis of ALS involves inflammation, oxidative stress, apoptosis, dysfunction of mitochondria, aggregation of SOD1 protein, and dysfunction of astroglia, which include a severe loss of EAAT2 in both the motor cortex and spinal cord [244, 245]. Additionally, several mouse models of ALS exhibit marked loss or inactivation of glutamate transporters [246]. Moreover, selective loss of EAAT2 has also been demonstrated in both sporadic and familial cases of ALS [247]. However, a large-scale clinical trial testing the efficacy of ceftriaxone (an EAAT2 expression enhancer) in ALS patients reported no significant difference in survival between placebo- and ceftriaxone-treated patients [248].

While glutamate transport dysfunction and excitotoxicity may contribute to the late stage of ALS disease progression, there is no consistent evidence supporting EAAT2 as a primary factor in motor neuron degeneration in ALS. A study found that overexpression of GLT-1 in the cervical spinal cord of SOD1G93A mice with ALS did not protect motor neurons, preserve diaphragm function, or prolong animal survival, thus challenging the notion that EAAT2 is a primary factor in motor neuron degeneration in ALS [249]. It is thought that simultaneous targeting of calcium overload, endoplasmic reticulum stress, and mitochondrial dysfunction pathways may be necessary to halt ALS progression [250].

Huntington's disease (HD): HD is a devastating neurodegenerative disorder characterized by degeneration of multiple brain areas, involving dopamine, glutamate, and GABA neurotransmitter systems. It is caused by a mutated form of the huntingtin gene, resulting in the accumulation of mutant protein aggregates [251], resulting in oxidative stress, mitochondrial dysfunction, and excitotoxicity [252]. Reduced EAAT2 mRNA levels have been observed in HD patients [253], and transgenic mouse models, while increased GLT-1 expression can improve behavioral symptoms in HD mouse models [254]. Additionally, EAAT3 expression has been shown to be reduced in HD; however, this appears to be associated with issues with cysteine transport and oxidative stress rather than increases in extracellular glutamate concentration.

These studies suggest that alterations in EAAT2 and EAAT3 expression or function can influence the progression of Huntington's disease (HD). However, effective therapies for HD have yet to be discovered and developed [71, 255, 256].

Human idiopathic Parkinson's disease (PD): is a progressive neurodegenerative movement disorder characterized by the degeneration of dopaminergic neurons, leading to increased firing rates of glutamatergic excitatory projections to the substantia nigra [257]. This disturbance may contribute to glutamate-mediated excitotoxicity, exacerbating nigrostriatal degeneration in PD. Studies using unilateral 6-hydroxydopamine (6-OHDA) animal models of PD have demonstrated a link between disturbed glutamatergic neurotransmission and glutamate transporter functioning in the striatum. A study revealed posttranslational modifications on GLT-1, resulting in transporter trafficking by Nedd4-2 in a PD model. Additionally, rapamycin protects mice against 1-methyl-4-phenyl-1,2,3,6-tetrahydropyridine (MPTP)-induced loss of dopaminergic neurons in a PD model, through preservation of EAAT2, an effect mediated by NF-κB. Moreover, it was reported that increased expression of GLT-1 with ceftriaxone ameliorated locomotor impairments in a PD model [258].

Dyskinesias are a motor complication that develops as common side effect of current PD treatments such as L-DOPA (L-3,4-dihydroxyphenylalanine), which is used to replenish dopamine levels. Dyskinesias are linked to elevated extracellular glutamate levels in the basal ganglia, thus targeting EAAT2 modulation may represent a potential therapeutic target to treat them.

Collectively, it seems that dysregulation or loss of EAATs function, especially, EAAT2, can lead to glutamatergic excitotoxicity and neuronal death, contributing to neurodegenerative diseases such as AD, ALS, HD, and PD. However, our current understanding of the contribution of EAATs in these diseases is primarily based on experimental models and post-mortem brain tissue analysis. Detecting EAAT2 in living human brains could greatly improve diagnosis and therapy for these neurodegenerative disorders, and this could allow the possibility of utilizing EAAT2 activation for therapeutic interventions.

3.10 Other disorders

HIV-associated neurocognitive disorder (HAND): A common neuropathology observed in the brains of HIV-infected individuals is the excess release of glutamate upon HIV infection of macrophage/microglial cells [71, 259]. This has been linked to neurotoxicity mediated by various HIV proteins, including gp120 and transactivator of transcription (TAT). NMDA receptor antagonists were not effective at mitigating glutamate excitotoxicity in HAND due to side effects. Therefore, alternative approaches are being pursued, such as modulating the activity or expression of glutamate transporters. A study found that methamphetamine and HIV treatment activate trace amine-associated receptor 1 (TAAR1) in human astrocytes, leading to reduced EAAT2 mRNA levels and impaired glutamate clearance. CCL2 impairs spatial memory and cognition, potentially through upregulating mRNA expression linked to inflammation, excitotoxicity, and neuronal apoptosis in HAND. However, our understanding of the host factors contributing to the neurotoxic effects of HIV-1 on the CNS is evolving, and identification of strategies to mitigate the neurotoxic effects of viral and host proteins is crucial to develop neuroprotection strategies to alleviate the detrimental impact of HIV-1 on the brain.

Autism: The etiology of autism spectrum disorder is complex and involves genetic predisposition, environmental influences, and other yet unknown factors. It is thought that glutamate excitotoxicity, mitochondrial dysfunction, and degeneration are key components of autism. A report by the Autism Genome Project Consortium identified a linkage peak for autism in the region of chromosome 11, where the gene for EAAT2 is situated [260]. There is evidence suggesting astroglial dysfunction in the autistic brain and activators of GLT-1 expression have been shown to ameliorate certain symptoms of autism and reduce epilepsy seizures, suggesting that GLT-1 may be a novel therapeutic strategy for autism.

Additionally, EAAT2 dysfunction has been implicated in the pathogenesis of major depressive disorders [261], mood disorders [262, 263], glioma [264, 265], multiple sclerosis [266], and schizophrenia [267], among others. Dysfunction of EAAT3 has also been observed in schizophrenia [13] and OCD [268].

Collectively, these studies suggest that therapies aimed at the modulation of the function and/or expression of EAATs, particularly EAAT2, could have broad therapeutic potential for various CNS disorders.

4. Conclusions

EAATs are key proteins that regulate the excitatory tone in CNS and are important for many physiological functions. Dysfunction in their activity or expression has profound effects that have been implicated in the etiology of many acute and chronic pathologies. In the past decade, it has become evident that drugs targeting NMDA receptors and secondary damages from glutamate-mediated excitotoxicity are limited and ineffective, often resulting in unwanted side effects; thus, there is a need for better therapeutics. In this regard, enhancing glutamate transporter expression or function pharmacologically holds great promise for therapeutic interventions, particularly targeting EAAT2 [71, 269].

Drug development targeting EAATs started with the discovery of pharmacological agents that were developed to study the intrinsic properties and function of the EAATs, specifically the potent EAAT2 inhibitors TBOA and analogs [68, 71]. TBOA was the first non-transportable blocker for all subtypes of EAATs identified, which helped elucidate several functions of the EAATs, and encouraged the search for other modulators of the function of EAATs. However, there is also a need to identify subtype-selective enhancers and inhibitors for all subtypes of glutamate transporters, to fully understand how to fine-tune the extracellular concentration of glutamate in the CNS. Several EAAT2 PAMs have already been identified, which can be administered acutely and thus are advantageous over the expression enhancers that generally require prophylactic administration. It is yet to be established whether small molecule allosteric activators of EAAT2, like many biologics, can undergo traditional pharmacokinetic analysis and demonstrate efficacy in animal models of CNS disease. The future may uncover whether this class of compounds is effective in chronic conditions and when used in combination therapies. Moreover, the recent publication of cryo-EM structures of EAAT2 presents an opportunity to launch a structural-based drug design initiative aimed at screening and developing high-affinity EAAT2 PAMs. These compounds can have therapeutic potential and serve as imaging tools to detect changes in EAAT2 density in neurodegenerative diseases. Furthermore, the optimal timing for therapeutic intervention with EAAT2-targeting drugs remains uncertain. Hence, discovering noninvasive methods to enhance our understanding of EAAT2 function and expression in the living brain is imperative. Finally, there is still more to understand about the molecular behavior of glutamate transporters in dysfunctions. Current understanding suggests that a complex process is involved in the down-regulation, reversal, and post-translational modifications of EAATs. The intracellular signaling pathways that accompany the changes in EAATs on disease states also need to be further understood.

In conclusion, EAAT dysfunction plays a significant role in many neuropsychiatric disorders. Recent advancements have propelled the pursuit of targeting these transporters as a strategy to prevent and treat glutamatergic dysfunctions. However, the full potential of modulating these transporters as a therapeutic target is yet to be fully understood, appreciated, and explored. We expect to see, in the upcoming years, the identification of an arsenal of selective pharmacological compounds that target these fascinating proteins and the investigation of their translational possibilities [71, 210].

Acknowledgements

ACKF received funding from NIH (RO1 NS111767), and KLR received financial support from the PhRMA foundation.

Conflict of interest

The authors declare no conflict of interest.

Author details

Katelyn L. Reeb, Simran K. Gill, Rhea Temmermand and Andréia C.K. Fontana*
Department of Pharmacology and Physiology, Drexel University College of Medicine, Philadelphia, PA, USA

*Address all correspondence to: acm83@drexel

References

[1] Olney JW. Brain lesions, obesity, and other disturbances in mice treated with monosodium glutamate. Science. 1969;**164**(3880):719-721

[2] Danbolt NC. Glutamate uptake. Progress in Neurobiology. 2001;**65**(1):1-105

[3] Lewerenz J, Hewett SJ, Huang Y, Lambros M, Gout PW, Kalivas PW, et al. The cystine/glutamate antiporter system x(c)(−) in health and disease: From molecular mechanisms to novel therapeutic opportunities. Antioxidants & Redox Signaling. 2013;**18**(5):522-555

[4] El Mestikawy S, Wallén-Mackenzie A, Fortin GM, Descarries L, Trudeau LE. From glutamate co-release to vesicular synergy: Vesicular glutamate transporters. Nature Reviews Neuroscience. 2011;**12**(4):204-216

[5] Roberts RC, Roche JK, McCullumsmith RE. Localization of excitatory amino acid transporters EAAT1 and EAAT2 in human postmortem cortex: A light and electron microscopic study. Neuroscience. 2014;**277**:522-540

[6] Pajarillo E, Rizor A, Lee J, Aschner M, Lee E. The role of astrocytic glutamate transporters GLT-1 and GLAST in neurological disorders: Potential targets for neurotherapeutics. Neuropharmacology. 2019;**161**:107559-107573

[7] Storck T, Schulte S, Hofmann K, Stoffel W. Structure, expression, and functional analysis of a Na(+)-dependent glutamate/aspartate transporter from rat brain. Proceedings of the National Academy of Sciences of the United States of America. 1992;**89**(22):10955-10959

[8] Suchak SK, Baloyianni NV, Perkinton MS, Williams RJ, Meldrum BS, Rattray M. The 'glial' glutamate transporter, EAAT2 (Glt-1) accounts for high affinity glutamate uptake into adult rodent nerve endings. Journal of Neurochemistry. 2003;**84**(3):522-532

[9] Pines G, Danbolt NC, Bjoras M, Zhang Y, Bendahan A, Eide L, et al. Cloning and expression of a rat brain L-glutamate transporter. Nature. 1992;**360**(6403):464-467

[10] Haugeto O, Ullensvang K, Levy LM, Chaudhry FA, Honore T, Nielsen M, et al. Brain glutamate transporter proteins form homomultimers. The Journal of Biological Chemistry. 1996;**271**(44):27715-27722

[11] Gegelashvili G, Danbolt NC, Schousboe A. Neuronal soluble factors differentially regulate the expression of the GLT1 and GLAST glutamate transporters in cultured astroglia. Journal of Neurochemistry. 1997;**69**(6):2612-2615

[12] Peacey E, Miller CC, Dunlop J, Rattray M. The four major N- and C-terminal splice variants of the excitatory amino acid transporter GLT-1 form cell surface homomeric and heteromeric assemblies. Molecular Pharmacology. 2009;**75**(5):1062-1073

[13] Bjorn-Yoshimoto WE, Underhill SM. The importance of the excitatory amino acid transporter 3 (EAAT3). Neurochemistry International. 2016;**98**:4-18

[14] Perkins EM, Clarkson YL, Suminaite D, Lyndon AR, Tanaka K, Rothstein JD, et al. Loss of cerebellar glutamate transporters EAAT4 and GLAST differentially affects the

spontaneous firing pattern and survival of Purkinje cells. Human Molecular Genetics. 2018;**27**(15):2614-2627

[15] Arriza JL, Eliasof S, Kavanaugh MP, Amara SG. Excitatory amino acid transporter 5, a retinal glutamate transporter coupled to a chloride conductance. Proceedings of the National Academy of Sciences of the United States of America. 1997;**94**(8):4155-4160

[16] Alleva C, Machtens JP, Kortzak D, Weyand I, Fahlke C. Molecular basis of coupled transport and anion conduction in excitatory amino acid transporters. Neurochemical Research. 2022;**47**(1):9-22

[17] Kosugi T, Kawahara K. Reversed actrocytic GLT-1 during ischemia is crucial to excitotoxic death of neurons, but contributes to the survival of astrocytes themselves. Neurochemical Research. 2006;**31**(7):933-943

[18] Ewers D, Becher T, Machtens JP, Weyand I, Fahlke C. Induced fit substrate binding to an archeal glutamate transporter homologue. Proceedings of the National Academy of Sciences of the United States of America. 2013;**110**(30):12486-12491

[19] Rose EM, Koo JC, Antflick JE, Ahmed SM, Angers S, Hampson DR. Glutamate transporter coupling to Na, K-ATPase. The Journal of Neuroscience. 2009;**29**(25):8143-8155

[20] Reyes N, Ginter C, Boudker O. Transport mechanism of a bacterial homologue of glutamate transporters. Nature. 2009;**462**(7275):880-885

[21] Akyuz N, Altman RB, Blanchard SC, Boudker O. Transport dynamics in a glutamate transporter homologue. Nature. 2013;**502**(7469):114-118

[22] Machtens JP, Kortzak D, Lansche C, Leinenweber A, Kilian P, Begemann B, et al. Mechanisms of anion conduction by coupled glutamate transporters. Cell. 2015;**160**(3):542-553

[23] Bergles DE, Tzingounis AV, Jahr CE. Comparison of coupled and uncoupled currents during glutamate uptake by GLT-1 transporters. The Journal of Neuroscience. 2002;**22**(23):10153

[24] Billups B, Rossi D, Attwell D. Anion conductance behavior of the glutamate uptake carrier in salamander retinal glial cells. The Journal of Neuroscience. 1996;**16**(21):6722-6731

[25] Winter N, Kovermann P, Fahlke C. A point mutation associated with episodic ataxia 6 increases glutamate transporter anion currents. Brain. 2012;**135**(Pt 11):3416-3425

[26] Canul-Tec JC, Assal R, Cirri E, Legrand P, Brier S, Chamot-Rooke J, et al. Structure and allosteric inhibition of excitatory amino acid transporter 1. Nature. 2017;**544**(7651):446-451

[27] Qiu B, Matthies D, Fortea E, Yu Z, Boudker O. Cryo-EM structures of excitatory amino acid transporter 3 visualize coupled substrate, sodium, and proton binding and transport. Science Advances. 2021;**7**(10):eabf5814

[28] Kato T, Kusakizako T, Jin C, Zhou X, Ohgaki R, Quan L, et al. Structural insights into inhibitory mechanism of human excitatory amino acid transporter EAAT2. Nature Communications. 2022;**13**(1):4714

[29] Zhang Z, Chen H, Geng Z, Yu Z, Li H, Dong Y, et al. Structural basis of ligand binding modes of human EAAT2. Nature Communications. 2022;**13**(1):3329

[30] Zhang C, Raghupathi R, Saatman KE, Smith DH, Stutzmann JM, Wahl F, et al. Riluzole attenuates cortical lesion size, but not hippocampal neuronal loss, following traumatic brain injury in the rat. Journal of Neuroscience Research. 1998;**52**(3):342-349

[31] Azbill RD, Mu X, Springer JE. Riluzole increases high-affinity glutamate uptake in rat spinal cord synaptosomes. Brain Research. 2000;**871**(2):175-180

[32] Mu X, Azbill RD, Springer JE. Riluzole and methylprednisolone combined treatment improves functional recovery in traumatic spinal cord injury. Journal of Neurotrauma. 2000;**17**(9):773-780

[33] Brothers HM, Bardou I, Hopp SC, Kaercher RM, Corona AW, Fenn AM, et al. Riluzole partially rescues age-associated, but not LPS-induced, loss of glutamate transporters and spatial memory. Journal of Neuroimmune Pharmacology. 2013;**8**(5):1098-1105

[34] Miller RG, Mitchell JD, Moore DH. Riluzole for amyotrophic lateral sclerosis (ALS)/motor neuron disease (MND). The Cochrane Database of Systematic Reviews. 2000;**2**(2):CD001447

[35] Frizzo ME, Dall'Onder LP, Dalcin KB, Souza DO. Riluzole enhances glutamate uptake in rat astrocyte cultures. Cellular and Molecular Neurobiology. 2004;**24**(1):123-128

[36] Fumagalli E, Funicello M, Rauen T, Gobbi M, Mennini T. Riluzole enhances the activity of glutamate transporters GLAST, GLT1 and EAAC1. European Journal of Pharmacology. 2008;**578**(2-3):171-176

[37] Banasr M, Chowdhury GM, Terwilliger R, Newton SS, Duman RS, Behar KL, et al. Glial pathology in an animal model of depression: Reversal of stress-induced cellular, metabolic and behavioral deficits by the glutamate-modulating drug riluzole. Molecular Psychiatry. 2010;**15**(5):501-511

[38] Carbone M, Duty S, Rattray M. Riluzole elevates GLT-1 activity and levels in striatal astrocytes. Neurochemistry International. 2012;**60**(1):31-38

[39] Wilson JR, Fehlings MG. Riluzole for acute traumatic spinal cord injury: A promising neuroprotective treatment strategy. World Neurosurgery. 2014;**81**(5-6):825-829

[40] Waibel S, Reuter A, Malessa S, Blaugrund E, Ludolph AC. Rasagiline alone and in combination with riluzole prolongs survival in an ALS mouse model. Journal of Neurology. 2004;**251**(9):1080-1084

[41] Del Signore SJ, Amante DJ, Kim J, Stack EC, Goodrich S, Cormier K, et al. Combined riluzole and sodium phenylbutyrate therapy in transgenic amyotrophic lateral sclerosis mice. Amyotrophic Lateral Sclerosis. 2009;**10**(2):85-94

[42] Whitcomb DJ, Molnar E. Is riluzole a new drug for Alzheimer's disease? Journal of Neurochemistry. 2015;**135**(2):207-209

[43] Al-Horani RA. Riluzole and its prodrugs for the treatment of Alzheimer's disease. Pharmaceutical Patent Analyst. 2023;**12**(2):79-85

[44] Fontana AC, Guizzo R, de Oliveira BR, Meirelles ESAR, Coimbra NC, Amara SG, et al. Purification of a neuroprotective component of Parawixia bistriata spider venom that enhances glutamate uptake. British Journal of Pharmacology. 2003;**139**(7):1297-1309

[45] Duffield M, Patel A, Mortensen OV, Schnur D, Gonzalez-Suarez AD, Torres-Salazar D, et al. Transport rate of EAAT2 is regulated by amino acid located at the interface between the scaffolding and substrate transport domains. Neurochemistry International. 2020;**139**:104792

[46] Kortagere S, Mortensen OV, Xia J, Lester W, Fang Y, Srikanth YVV, et al. Identification of novel allosteric modulators of glutamate transporter EAAT2. ACS Chemical Neuroscience. 2017;**9**(3):522-534

[47] Forster YM, Green JL, Khatiwada A, Liberato JL, Reddy PAN, Salvino JM, et al. Elucidation of the structure and synthesis of neuroprotective low molecular mass components of the *Parawixia bistriata* spider venom. ACS Chemical Neuroscience. 2020;**11**(11):1573-1596

[48] Fachim HA, Mortari MR, Gobbo-Netto L, Dos Santos WF. Neuroprotective activity of parawixin 10, a compound isolated from *Parawixia bistriata* spider venom (Araneidae: Araneae) in rats undergoing intrahippocampal NMDA microinjection. Pharmacognosy Magazine. 2015;**11**(43):579-585

[49] Fachim HA, Cunha AO, Pereira AC, Beleboni RO, Gobbo-Neto L, Lopes NP, et al. Neurobiological activity of *Parawixin* 10, a novel anticonvulsant compound isolated from *Parawixia bistriata* spider venom (Araneidae: Araneae). Epilepsy & Behavior. 2011;**22**(2):158-164

[50] Liberato JL, Godoy LD, Mortari MR, Gobbo-Neto L, Lopes NP, Santos WF. Parawixin10: A new natural compound from *Parawixia bistriata* spider venom that presents neuroprotective, memory-saving, and disease-modifying effects in the pilocarpine model of TLE in Wistar rats. Epilepsy & Behavior. 2014;**38**:196

[51] Abram M, Jakubiec M, Reeb K, Cheng MH, Gedschold R, Rapacz A, et al. Discovery of (R)-N-benzyl-2-(2,5-dioxopyrrolidin-1-yl)propanamide [(R)-AS-1], a novel orally bioavailable EAAT2 modulator with drug-like properties and potent antiseizure activity *in vivo*. Journal of Medicinal Chemistry. 2022;**65**(17):11703-11725

[52] O'Shea RD, Fodera MV, Aprico K, Dehnes Y, Danbolt NC, Crawford D, et al. Evaluation of drugs acting at glutamate transporters in organotypic hippocampal cultures: New evidence on substrates and blockers in excitotoxicity. Neurochemical Research. 2002;**27**(1-2):5-13

[53] Lebrun B, Sakaitani M, Shimamoto K, Yasuda-Kamatani Y, Nakajima T. New beta-hydroxyaspartate derivatives are competitive blockers for the bovine glutamate/aspartate transporter. The Journal of Biological Chemistry. 1997;**272**(33):20336-20339

[54] Shimamoto K. Glutamate transporter blockers for elucidation of the function of excitatory neurotransmission systems. Chemical Record. 2008;**8**(3):182-199

[55] Shigeri Y, Seal RP, Shimamoto K. Molecular pharmacology of glutamate transporters, EAATs and VGLUTs. Brain Research. Brain Research Reviews. 2004;**45**(3):250-265

[56] Shimamoto K, Lebrun B, Yasuda-Kamatani Y, Sakaitani M, Shigeri Y, Yumoto N, et al. DL-threo-beta-benzyloxyaspartate, a potent blocker of excitatory amino acid transporters. Molecular Pharmacology. 1998;**53**(2):195-201

[57] Izumi Y, Shimamoto K, Benz AM, Hammerman SB, Olney JW,

Zorumski CF. Glutamate transporters and retinal excitotoxicity. GLIA. 2002;**39**(1):58-68

[58] Bonde C, Noraberg J, Noer H, Zimmer J. Ionotropic glutamate receptors and glutamate transporters are involved in necrotic neuronal cell death induced by oxygen-glucose deprivation of hippocampal slice cultures. Neuroscience. 2005;**136**(3):779-794

[59] Jabaudon D, Shimamoto K, Yasuda-Kamatani Y, Scanziani M, Gahwiler BH, Gerber U. Inhibition of uptake unmasks rapid extracellular turnover of glutamate of nonvesicular origin. Proceedings of the National Academy of Sciences of the United States of America. 1999;**96**(15):8733-8738

[60] Vandenberg RJ, Ryan RM. Mechanisms of glutamate transport. Physiological Reviews. 2013;**93**(4):1621-1657

[61] Shimamoto K, Sakai R, Takaoka K, Yumoto N, Nakajima T, Amara SG, et al. Characterization of novel L-threo-beta-benzyloxyaspartate derivatives, potent blockers of the glutamate transporters. Molecular Pharmacology. 2004;**65**(4):1008-1015

[62] Bozzo L, Chatton JY. Inhibitory effects of (2S, 3S)-3-[3-[4-(trifluoromethyl)benzoylamino] benzyloxy]aspartate (TFB-TBOA) on the astrocytic sodium responses to glutamate. Brain Research. 2010;**1316**:27-34

[63] Tsukada S, Iino M, Takayasu Y, Shimamoto K, Ozawa S. Effects of a novel glutamate transporter blocker, (2S, 3S)-3-[3-[4-(trifluoromethyl)benzoylamino] benzyloxy]aspartate (TFB-TBOA), on activities of hippocampal neurons. Neuropharmacology. 2005;**48**(4):479-491

[64] Martinez D, Rogers RC, Hermann GE, Hasser EM, Kline DD. Astrocytic glutamate transporters reduce the neuronal and physiological influence of metabotropic glutamate receptors in nucleus tractus solitarii. American Journal of Physiology. Regulatory, Integrative and Comparative Physiology. 2020;**318**(3):R545-Rr64

[65] Fontana ACK, Poli ANR, Gour J, Srikanth YVV, Anastasi N, Ashok D, et al. Synthesis and structure-activity relationships for glutamate transporter allosteric modulators. Journal of Medicinal Chemistry. 2024;**67**(8):6119-6143

[66] McIntosh TK, Smith DH, Voddi M, Perri BR, Stutzmann JM. Riluzole, a novel neuroprotective agent, attenuates both neurologic motor and cognitive dysfunction following experimental brain injury in the rat. Journal of Neurotrauma. 1996;**13**(12):767-780

[67] Abdel-Magid AF. Allosteric modulators: An emerging concept in drug discovery. ACS Medicinal Chemistry Letters. 2015;**6**(2):104-107

[68] Bridges RJ, Kavanaugh MP, Chamberlin AR. A pharmacological review of competitive inhibitors and substrates of high-affinity, sodium-dependent glutamate transport in the central nervous system. Current Pharmaceutical Design. 1999;**5**(5):363-379

[69] Niello M, Gradisch R, Loland CJ, Stockner T, Sitte HH. Allosteric modulation of neurotransmitter transporters as a therapeutic strategy. Trends in Pharmacological Sciences. 2020;**41**(7):446-463

[70] Anderson CM, Swanson RA. Astrocyte glutamate transport: Review of properties, regulation, and physiological functions. GLIA. 2000;**32**(1):1-14

[71] Fontana AC. Current approaches to enhance glutamate transporter function and expression. Journal of Neurochemistry. 2015;**134**(6):982-1007

[72] Rothstein JD, Patel S, Regan MR, Haenggeli C, Huang YH, Bergles DE, et al. Beta-lactam antibiotics offer neuroprotection by increasing glutamate transporter expression. Nature. 2005;**433**(7021):73-77

[73] Chu K, Lee ST, Sinn DI, Ko SY, Kim EH, Kim JM, et al. Pharmacological induction of ischemic tolerance by glutamate transporter-1 (EAAT2) upregulation. Stroke; a Journal of Cerebral Circulation. 2007;**38**(1):177-182

[74] Hu Y, Li W, Lu L, Cai J, Xian X, Zhang M, et al. An anti-nociceptive role for ceftriaxone in chronic neuropathic pain in rats. Pain. 2010;**148**(2):284-301

[75] Ramos KM, Lewis MT, Morgan KN, Crysdale NY, Kroll JL, Taylor FR, et al. Spinal upregulation of glutamate transporter GLT-1 by ceftriaxone: Therapeutic efficacy in a range of experimental nervous system disorders. Neuroscience. 2010;**169**(4):1888-1900

[76] Rao PS, Goodwani S, Bell RL, Wei Y, Boddu SH, Sari Y. Effects of ampicillin, cefazolin and cefoperazone treatments on GLT-1 expressions in the mesocorticolimbic system and ethanol intake in alcohol-preferring rats. Neuroscience. 2015;**295**:164-174

[77] Kim J, John J, Langford D, Walker E, Ward S, Rawls SM. Clavulanic acid enhances glutamate transporter subtype I (GLT-1) expression and decreases reinforcing efficacy of cocaine in mice. Amino Acids. 2016;**48**(3):689-696

[78] Melzer N, Meuth SG, Torres-Salazar D, Bittner S, Zozulya AL, Weidenfeller C, et al. A beta-lactam antibiotic dampens excitotoxic inflammatory CNS damage in a mouse model of multiple sclerosis. PLoS One. 2008;**3**(9):e3149

[79] Rawls SM, Karaca F, Madhani I, Bhojani V, Martinez RL, Abou-Gharbia M, et al. β-lactamase inhibitors display anti-seizure properties in an invertebrate assay. Neuroscience. 2010;**169**(4):1800-1804

[80] Rao PS, Saternos H, Goodwani S, Sari Y. Effects of ceftriaxone on GLT1 isoforms, xCT and associated signaling pathways in P rats exposed to ethanol. Psychopharmacology. 2015;**232**(13):2333-2342

[81] Lipski J, Wan CK, Bai JZ, Pi R, Li D, Donnelly D. Neuroprotective potential of ceftriaxone in *in vitro* models of stroke. Neuroscience. 2007;**146**(2):617-629

[82] Thone-Reineke C, Neumann C, Namsolleck P, Schmerbach K, Krikov M, Schefe JH, et al. The beta-lactam antibiotic, ceftriaxone, dramatically improves survival, increases glutamate uptake and induces neurotrophins in stroke. Journal of Hypertension. 2008;**26**(12):2426-2435

[83] Pan XD, Wei J, Xiao GM. Effects of beta-lactam antibiotics ceftriaxone on expression of glutamate in hippocampus after traumatic brain injury in rats. Zhejiang da xue xue bao Yi xue ban = Journal of Zhejiang University Medical sciences. 2011;**40**(5):522-526

[84] Wei J, Pan X, Pei Z, Wang W, Qiu W, Shi Z, et al. The beta-lactam antibiotic, ceftriaxone, provides neuroprotective potential via anti-excitotoxicity and anti-inflammation response in a rat model of traumatic brain injury. Journal of Trauma and Acute Care Surgery. 2012;**73**(3):654-660

[85] Cui C, Cui Y, Gao J, Sun L, Wang Y, Wang K, et al. Neuroprotective effect of ceftriaxone in a rat model of traumatic brain injury. Neurological Sciences. 2014;**35**(5):695-700

[86] Goodrich GS, Kabakov AY, Hameed MQ, Dhamne SC, Rosenberg PA, Rotenberg A. Ceftriaxone treatment after traumatic brain injury restores expression of the glutamate transporter, GLT-1, reduces regional gliosis, and reduces post-traumatic seizures in the rat. Journal of Neurotrauma. 2013;**30**(16):1434-1441

[87] Leung TC, Lui CN, Chen LW, Yung WH, Chan YS, Yung KK. Ceftriaxone ameliorates motor deficits and protects dopaminergic neurons in 6-hydroxydopamine-lesioned rats. ACS Chemical Neuroscience. 2012;**3**(1):22-30

[88] Kelsey JE, Neville C. The effects of the beta-lactam antibiotic, ceftriaxone, on forepaw stepping and L-DOPA-induced dyskinesia in a rodent model of Parkinson's disease. Psychopharmacology. 2014;**231**(12):2405-2415

[89] Miller BR, Dorner JL, Shou M, Sari Y, Barton SJ, Sengelaub DR, et al. Up-regulation of GLT1 expression increases glutamate uptake and attenuates the Huntington's disease phenotype in the R6/2 mouse. Neuroscience. 2008;**153**(1):329-337

[90] Rebec GV. Dysregulation of corticostriatal ascorbate release and glutamate uptake in transgenic models of Huntington's disease. Antioxidants & Redox Signaling. 2013;**19**(17):2115-2128

[91] Feng D, Wang W, Dong Y, Wu L, Huang J, Ma Y, et al. Ceftriaxone alleviates early brain injury after subarachnoid hemorrhage by increasing excitatory amino acid transporter 2 expression via the PI3K/Akt/NF-kappaB signaling pathway. Neuroscience. 2014;**268**:21-32

[92] Hu YY, Xu J, Zhang M, Wang D, Li L, Li WB. Ceftriaxone modulates uptake activity of glial glutamate transporter-1 against global brain ischemia in rats. Journal of Neurochemistry. 2015;**132**(2):194-205

[93] Jagadapillai R, Mellen NM, Sachleben LR Jr, Gozal E. Ceftriaxone preserves glutamate transporters and prevents intermittent hypoxia-induced vulnerability to brain excitotoxic injury. PLoS One. 2014;**9**(7):e100230

[94] Beghi E, Bendotti C, Mennini T. New ideas for therapy in ALS: Critical considerations. Amyotrophic Lateral Sclerosis. 2006;**7**(2):126-127; discussion 7

[95] Nederkoorn PJ, Westendorp WF, Hooijenga IJ, de Haan RJ, Dippel DW, Vermeij FH, et al. Preventive antibiotics in stroke study: Rationale and protocol for a randomised trial. International Journal of Stroke. 2011;**6**(2):159-163

[96] Berry JD, Shefner JM, Conwit R, Schoenfeld D, Keroack M, Felsenstein D, et al. Design and initial results of a multi-phase randomized trial of ceftriaxone in amyotrophic lateral sclerosis. PLoS One. 2013;**8**(4):e61177

[97] Cudkowicz M, Shefner J, Consortium N. STAGE 3 clinical trial of ceftriaxone in subjects with ALS (S36.001). Neurology. 2013;**80**:S36.001

[98] Hota SK, Barhwal K, Ray K, Singh SB, Ilavazhagan G. Ceftriaxone rescues hippocampal neurons from excitotoxicity and enhances memory retrieval in chronic hypobaric hypoxia. Neurobiology of Learning and Memory. 2008;**89**(4):522-532

[99] Lee SG, Su ZZ, Emdad L, Gupta P, Sarkar D, Borjabad A, et al. Mechanism of ceftriaxone induction of excitatory amino acid transporter-2 expression and glutamate uptake in primary human astrocytes. The Journal of Biological Chemistry. 2008;**283**(19):13116-13123

[100] Verma R, Mishra V, Sasmal D, Raghubir R. Pharmacological evaluation of glutamate transporter 1 (GLT-1) mediated neuroprotection following cerebral ischemia/reperfusion injury. European Journal of Pharmacology. 2010;**638**(1-3):65-71

[101] Kolahdouz M, Jafari F, Falanji F, Nazemi S, Mohammadzadeh M, Molavi M, et al. Clavulanic acid attenuating effect on the diabetic neuropathic pain in rats. Neurochemical Research. 2021;**46**(7):1759-1770

[102] Schroeder JA, Tolman NG, McKenna FF, Watkins KL, Passeri SM, Hsu AH, et al. Clavulanic acid reduces rewarding, hyperthermic and locomotor-sensitizing effects of morphine in rats: A new indication for an old drug? Drug and Alcohol Dependence. 2014;**142**:41-45

[103] Philogene-Khalid HL, Morrison MF, Darbinian N, Selzer ME, Schroeder J, Rawls SM. The GLT-1 enhancer clavulanic acid suppresses cocaine place preference behavior and reduces GCPII activity and protein levels in the rat nucleus accumbens. Drug and Alcohol Dependence. 2022;**232**:109306

[104] Ochoa-Aguilar A, Ventura-Martinez R, Sotomayor-Sobrino MA, Jaimez R, Coffeen U, Jiménez-González A, et al. Ceftriaxone and clavulanic acid induce antiallodynia and anti-inflammatory effects in rats using the carrageenan model. Journal of Pain Research. 2018;**11**:977-985

[105] Kristensen PJ, Gegelashvili G, Munro G, Heegaard AM, Bjerrum OJ. The β-lactam clavulanic acid mediates glutamate transport-sensitive pain relief in a rat model of neuropathic pain. European Journal of Pain. 2018;**22**(2):282-294

[106] Hajhashemi V, Dehdashti K. Antinociceptive effect of clavulanic acid and its preventive activity against development of morphine tolerance and dependence in animal models. Results in Pharma Sciences. 2014;**9**(5):315-321

[107] Kong Q, Chang L-C, Takahashi K, Liu Q, Schulte DA, Lai L, et al. Small-molecule activator of glutamate transporter EAAT2 translation provides neuroprotection. The Journal of Clinical Investigation. 2014;**124**(3):1255-1267

[108] Tejeda-Bayron FA, Rivera-Aponte DE, Malpica-Nieves CJ, Maldonado-Martinez G, Maldonado HM, Skatchkov SN, et al. Activation of glutamate transporter-1 (GLT-1) confers sex-dependent neuroprotection in brain ischemia. Brain Sciences. 2021;**11**(1):76

[109] Colton CK, Kong Q, Lai L, Zhu MX, Seyb KI, Cuny GD, et al. Identification of translational activators of glial glutamate transporter EAAT2 through cell-based high-throughput screening: An approach to prevent excitotoxicity. Journal of Biomolecular Screening. 2010;**15**(6):653-662

[110] Xing X, Chang LC, Kong Q, Colton CK, Lai L, Glicksman MA, et al. Structure-activity relationship study of pyridazine derivatives as glutamate transporter EAAT2 activators. Bioorganic & Medicinal Chemistry Letters. 2011;**21**(19):5774-5777

[111] Takahashi K, Kong Q, Lin Y, Stouffer N, Schulte DA, Lai L, et al. Restored glial glutamate transporter EAAT2 function as a potential therapeutic approach for Alzheimer's

disease. The Journal of Experimental Medicine. 2015;**212**(3):319-332

[112] Alotaibi G, Rahman S. Effects of glial glutamate transporter activator in formalin-induced pain behaviour in mice. European Journal of Pain (London, England). 2019;**23**(4):765-783

[113] Mao QX, Yang TD. Amitriptyline upregulates EAAT1 and EAAT2 in neuropathic pain rats. Brain Research Bulletin. 2010;**81**(4-5):424-427

[114] Moore RA, Derry S, Aldington D, Cole P, Wiffen PJ. Amitriptyline for neuropathic pain in adults. The Cochrane Database of Systematic Reviews. 2015;**2015**(7):Cd008242

[115] Krzyzanowska W, Pomierny B, Bystrowska B, Pomierny-Chamiolo L, Filip M, Budziszewska B, et al. Ceftriaxone- and N-acetylcysteine-induced brain tolerance to ischemia: Influence on glutamate levels in focal cerebral ischemia. PLoS One. 2017;**12**(10):e0186243

[116] Oka S, Kamata H, Kamata K, Yagisawa H, Hirata H. N-acetylcysteine suppresses TNF-induced NF-kappaB activation through inhibition of IkappaB kinases. FEBS Letters. 2000;**472**(2-3):196-202

[117] Sitcheran R, Gupta P, Fisher PB, Baldwin AS. Positive and negative regulation of EAAT2 by NF-kappaB: A role for N-myc in TNFalpha-controlled repression. The EMBO Journal. 2005;**24**(3):510-520

[118] Jastrzębska J, Frankowska M, Filip M, Atlas D. N-acetylcysteine amide (AD4) reduces cocaine-induced reinstatement. Psychopharmacology. 2016;**233**(18):3437-3448

[119] Ramirez-Niño AM, D'Souza MS, Markou A. N-acetylcysteine decreased nicotine self-administration and cue-induced reinstatement of nicotine seeking in rats: Comparison with the effects of N-acetylcysteine on food responding and food seeking. Psychopharmacology. 2013;**225**(2):473-482

[120] Quintanilla ME, Rivera-Meza M, Berríos-Cárcamo P, Salinas-Luypaert C, Herrera-Marschitz M, Israel Y. Beyond the "First Hit": Marked inhibition by N-acetyl cysteine of chronic ethanol intake but not of early ethanol intake. Parallel effects on ethanol-induced saccharin motivation. Alcoholism, Clinical and Experimental Research. 2016;**40**(5):1044-1051

[121] Reissner KJ, Gipson CD, Tran PK, Knackstedt LA, Scofield MD, Kalivas PW. Glutamate transporter GLT-1 mediates N-acetylcysteine inhibition of cocaine reinstatement. Addiction Biology. 2015;**20**(2):316-323

[122] Nie H, Zhang H, Weng HR. Minocycline prevents impaired glial glutamate uptake in the spinal sensory synapses of neuropathic rats. Neuroscience. 2010;**170**(3):901-912

[123] Sheldon AL, Gonzalez MI, Krizman-Genda EN, Susarla BT, Robinson MB. Ubiquitination-mediated internalization and degradation of the astroglial glutamate transporter, GLT-1. Neurochemistry International. 2008;**53**(6-8):296-308

[124] Park HJ, Baik HJ, Kim DY, Lee GY, Woo JH, Zuo Z, et al. Doxepin and imipramine but not fluoxetine reduce the activity of the rat glutamate transporter EAAT3 expressed in Xenopus oocytes. BMC Anesthesiology. 2015;**15**:116

[125] Susarla BT, Robinson MB. Internalization and degradation of the glutamate transporter GLT-1 in response

to phorbol ester. Neurochemistry International. 2008;**52**(4-5):709-722

[126] Dowd LA, Robinson MB. Rapid stimulation of EAAC1-mediated Na+–dependent L-glutamate transport activity in C6 glioma cells by phorbol ester. Journal of Neurochemistry. 1996;**67**(2):508-516

[127] Davis KE, Straff DJ, Weinstein EA, Bannerman PG, Correale DM, Rothstein JD, et al. Multiple signaling pathways regulate cell surface expression and activity of the excitatory amino acid carrier 1 subtype of Glu transporter in C6 glioma. The Journal of Neuroscience. 1998;**18**(7):2475-2485

[128] Ryan RM, Ingram SL, Scimemi A. Regulation of glutamate, GABA and dopamine transporter uptake, surface mobility and expression. Frontiers in Cellular Neuroscience. 2021;**15**:670346

[129] Gregg RA, Hicks C, Nayak SU, Tallarida CS, Nucero P, Smith GR, et al. Synthetic cathinone MDPV downregulates glutamate transporter subtype I (GLT-1) and produces rewarding and locomotor-activating effects that are reduced by a GLT-1 activator. Neuropharmacology. 2016;**108**:111-119

[130] Underhill SM, Wheeler DS, Li M, Watts SD, Ingram SL, Amara SG. Amphetamine modulates glutamatergic neurotransmission through endocytosis of the excitatory amino acid transporter EAAT3 in dopamine neurons. Neuron. 2014;**83**(2):404-416

[131] Li M-H, Underhill SM, Reed C, Phillips TJ, Amara SG, Ingram SL. Amphetamine and methamphetamine increase NMDAR-GluN2B synaptic currents in midbrain dopamine neurons. Neuropsychopharmacology. 2017;**42**(7):1539-1547

[132] Grewer C, Gameiro A, Rauen T. SLC1 glutamate transporters. Pflügers Archiv. 2014;**466**(1):3-24

[133] Conradt M, Stoffel W. Inhibition of the high-affinity brain glutamate transporter GLAST-1 via direct phosphorylation. Journal of Neurochemistry. 1997;**68**(3):1244-1251

[134] Gegelashvili G, Dehnes Y, Danbolt NC, Schousboe A. The high-affinity glutamate transporters GLT1, GLAST, and EAAT4 are regulated via different signalling mechanisms. Neurochemistry International. 2000;**37**(2-3):163-170

[135] Karki P, Smith K, Johnson J Jr, Aschner M, Lee EY. Genetic dys-regulation of astrocytic glutamate transporter EAAT2 and its implications in neurological disorders and manganese toxicity. Neurochemical Research. 2015;**40**(2):380-388

[136] Peterson AR, Binder DK. Post-translational regulation of GLT-1 in neurological diseases and its potential as an effective therapeutic target. Frontiers in Molecular Neuroscience. 2019;**12**:164

[137] Huang K, Kang MH, Askew C, Kang R, Sanders SS, Wan J, et al. Palmitoylation and function of glial glutamate transporter-1 is reduced in the YAC128 mouse model of Huntington disease. Neurobiology of Disease. 2010;**40**(1):207-215

[138] Foran E, Rosenblum L, Bogush A, Pasinelli P, Trotti D. Sumoylation of the astroglial glutamate transporter EAAT2 governs its intracellular compartmentalization. GLIA. 2014;**62**(8):1241-1253

[139] Szatkowski M, Barbour B, Attwell D. Non-vesicular release of glutamate from glial cells by reversed

electrogenic glutamate uptake. Nature. 1990;**348**(6300):443-446

[140] Katayama Y, Becker DP, Tamura T, Hovda DA. Massive increases in extracellular potassium and the indiscriminate release of glutamate following concussive brain injury. Journal of Neurosurgery. 1990;**73**(6):889-900

[141] Phillis JW, O'Regan MH. Mechanisms of glutamate and aspartate release in the ischemic rat cerebral cortex. Brain Research. 1996;**730**(1-2):150-164

[142] Volterra A, Trotti D, Tromba C, Floridi S, Racagni G. Glutamate uptake inhibition by oxygen free radicals in rat cortical astrocytes. The Journal of Neuroscience. 1994;**14**(5 Pt 1):2924-2932

[143] Rothstein JD. Excitotoxicity and neurodegeneration in amyotrophic lateral sclerosis. Clinical Neuroscience. 1995;**3**(6):348-359

[144] Lipton SA. Failures and successes of NMDA receptor antagonists: Molecular basis for the use of open-channel blockers like memantine in the treatment of acute and chronic neurologic insults. NeuroRx. 2004;**1**(1):101-110

[145] Tanaka K, Watase K, Manabe T, Yamada K, Watanabe M, Takahashi K, et al. Epilepsy and exacerbation of brain injury in mice lacking the glutamate transporter GLT-1. Science. 1997;**276**(5319):1699-1702

[146] Hakuba N, Koga K, Gyo K, Usami SI, Tanaka K. Exacerbation of noise-induced hearing loss in mice lacking the glutamate transporter GLAST. The Journal of Neuroscience. 2000;**20**(23):8750-8753

[147] Rao VL, Baskaya MK, Dogan A, Rothstein JD, Dempsey RJ. Traumatic brain injury down-regulates glial glutamate transporter (GLT-1 and GLAST) proteins in rat brain. Journal of Neurochemistry. 1998;**70**(5):2020-2027

[148] Matsugami TR, Tanemura K, Mieda M, Nakatomi R, Yamada K, Kondo T, et al. From the Cover: Indispensability of the glutamate transporters GLAST and GLT1 to brain development. Proceedings of the National Academy of Sciences of the United States of America. 2006;**103**(32):12161-12166

[149] Rothstein JD, Dykes-Hoberg M, Pardo CA, Bristol LA, Jin L, Kuncl RW, et al. Knockout of glutamate transporters reveals a major role for astroglial transport in excitotoxicity and clearance of glutamate. Neuron. 1996;**16**(3):675-686

[150] Barnett NL, Pow DV. Antisense knockdown of GLAST, a glial glutamate transporter, compromises retinal function. Investigative Ophthalmology & Visual Science. 2000;**41**(2):585-591

[151] Karlsson RM, Adermark L, Molander A, Perreau-Lenz S, Singley E, Solomon M, et al. Reduced alcohol intake and reward associated with impaired endocannabinoid signaling in mice with a deletion of the glutamate transporter GLAST. Neuropharmacology. 2012;**63**(2):181-189

[152] Peghini P, Janzen J, Stoffel W. Glutamate transporter EAAC-1-deficient mice develop dicarboxylic aminoaciduria and behavioral abnormalities but no neurodegeneration. The EMBO Journal. 1997;**16**(13):3822-3832

[153] Aoyama K, Suh SW, Hamby AM, Liu J, Chan WY, Chen Y, et al. Neuronal glutathione deficiency and age-dependent neurodegeneration in

the EAAC1 deficient mouse. Nature Neuroscience. 2006;**9**(1):119-126

[154] Watts SD, Torres-Salazar D, Divito CB, Amara SG. Cysteine transport through excitatory amino acid transporter 3 (EAAT3). PLoS One. 2014;**9**(10):e109245

[155] Bailey CG, Ryan RM, Thoeng AD, Ng C, King K, Vanslambrouck JM, et al. Loss-of-function mutations in the glutamate transporter SLC1A1 cause human dicarboxylic aminoaciduria. The Journal of Clinical Investigation. 2011;**121**(1):446-453

[156] Nikkuni O, Takayasu Y, Iino M, Tanaka K, Ozawa S. Facilitated activation of metabotropic glutamate receptors in cerebellar Purkinje cells in glutamate transporter EAAT4-deficient mice. Neuroscience Research. 2007;**59**(3):296-303

[157] Lukasiewcz PD, Bligard GW, DeBrecht JD. EAAT5 glutamate transporter-mediated inhibition in the vertebrate retina. Frontiers in Cellular Neuroscience. 2021;**15**:662859

[158] Beresford IJ, Parsons AA, Hunter AJ. Treatments for stroke. Expert Opinion on Emerging Drugs. 2003;**8**(1):103-122

[159] Puig B, Brenna S, Magnus T. Molecular communication of a dying neuron in stroke. International Journal of Molecular Sciences. 2018;**19**(9):2834

[160] Wetterling F, Chatzikonstantinou E, Tritschler L, Meairs S, Fatar M, Schad LR. Investigating potentially salvageable penumbra tissue in an *in vivo* model of transient ischemic stroke using sodium, diffusion, and perfusion magnetic resonance imaging. BMC Neuroscience. 2016;**17**(1):82

[161] Krzyzanowska W, Pomierny B, Filip M, Pera J. Glutamate transporters in brain ischemia: To modulate or not? Acta Pharmacologica Sinica. 2014;**35**(4):444-462

[162] Levy LM, Lehre KP, Walaas SI, Storm-Mathisen J, Danbolt NC. Down-regulation of glial glutamate transporters after glutamatergic denervation in the rat brain. The European Journal of Neuroscience. 1995;**7**(10):2036-2041

[163] Dong X, Wang Y, Qin Z. Molecular mechanisms of excitotoxicity and their relevance to pathogenesis of neurodegenerative diseases. Acta Pharmacologica Sinica. 2009;**30**:379-387

[164] Wu HY, Tomizawa K, Oda Y, Wei FY, Lu YF, Matsushita M, et al. Critical role of calpain-mediated cleavage of calcineurin in excitotoxic neurodegeneration. The Journal of Biological Chemistry. 2004;**279**(6):4929-4940

[165] Beckman JS, Chen J, Crow JP, Ye YZ. Reactions of nitric oxide, superoxide and peroxynitrite with superoxide dismutase in neurodegeneration. Progress in Brain Research. 1994;**103**:371-380

[166] Shen Y, Lu H, Xu R, Tian H, Xia X, Zhou FH, et al. The expression of GLAST and GLT1 in a transient cerebral ischemia Mongolian gerbil model. Neuropsychiatric Disease and Treatment. 2020;**16**:789-800

[167] Wang D, Zhao Y, Zhang Y, Zhang T, Shang X, Wang J, et al. Hypothermia protects against oxygen-glucose deprivation-induced neuronal injury by down-regulating the reverse transport of glutamate by astrocytes as mediated by neurons. Neuroscience. 2013;**237**:130-138

[168] Al Awabdh S, Gupta-Agarwal S, Sheehan DF, Muir J, Norkett R, Twelvetrees AE, et al. Neuronal activity mediated regulation of glutamate

transporter GLT-1 surface diffusion in rat astrocytes in dissociated and slice cultures. GLIA. 2016;**64**(7):1252-1264

[169] Abulseoud OA, Alasmari F, Hussein AM, Sari Y. Ceftriaxone as a novel therapeutic agent for hyperglutamatergic states: Bridging the gap between preclinical results and clinical translation. Frontiers in Neuroscience. 2022;**16**:841036

[170] Palmer AM, Marion DW, Botscheller ML, Swedlow PE, Styren SD, DeKosky ST. Traumatic brain injury-induced excitotoxicity assessed in a controlled cortical impact model. Journal of Neurochemistry. 1993;**61**(6):2015-2024

[171] Ikematsu K, Tsuda R, Kondo T, Nakasono I. The expression of excitatory amino acid transporter 2 in traumatic brain injury. Forensic Science International. 2002;**130**(2-3):83-89

[172] Rao VL, Dogan A, Bowen KK, Todd KG, Dempsey RJ. Antisense knockdown of the glial glutamate transporter GLT-1 exacerbates hippocampal neuronal damage following traumatic injury to rat brain. The European Journal of Neuroscience. 2001;**13**(1):119-128

[173] Collins M, Lovell MR, Iverson GL, Ide T, Maroon J. Examining concussion rates and return to play in high school football players wearing newer helmet technology: A three-year prospective cohort study. Neurosurgery. 2006;**58**(2):275-286; discussion-86

[174] Matute C, Domercq M, Sanchez-Gomez MV. Glutamate-mediated glial injury: Mechanisms and clinical importance. GLIA. 2006;**53**(2):212-224

[175] Jabs R, Seifert G, Steinhauser C. Astrocytic function and its alteration in the epileptic brain. Epilepsia. 2008;**49**(Suppl. 2):3-12

[176] Green JL, Dos Santos WF, Fontana ACK. Role of glutamate excitotoxicity and glutamate transporter EAAT2 in epilepsy: Opportunities for novel therapeutics development. Biochemical Pharmacology. 2021;**193**:114786

[177] Coutinho-Netto J, Abdul-Ghani AS, Collins JF, Bradford HF. Is glutamate a trigger factor in epileptic hyperactivity? Epilepsia. 1981;**22**(3):289-296

[178] Petr GT, Sun Y, Frederick NM, Zhou Y, Dhamne SC, Hameed MQ, et al. Conditional deletion of the glutamate transporter GLT-1 reveals that astrocytic GLT-1 protects against fatal epilepsy while neuronal GLT-1 contributes significantly to glutamate uptake into synaptosomes. The Journal of Neuroscience. 2015;**35**(13):5187-5201

[179] During MJ, Spencer DD. Extracellular hippocampal glutamate and spontaneous seizure in the conscious human brain. Lancet. 1993;**341**(8861):1607-1610

[180] Mathern GW, Mendoza D, Lozada A, Pretorius JK, Dehnes Y, Danbolt NC, et al. Hippocampal GABA and glutamate transporter immunoreactivity in patients with temporal lobe epilepsy. Neurology. 1999;**52**(3):453-472

[181] Lopes MW, Soares FM, de Mello N, Nunes JC, Cajado AG, de Brito D, et al. Time-dependent modulation of AMPA receptor phosphorylation and mRNA expression of NMDA receptors and glial glutamate transporters in the rat hippocampus and cerebral cortex in a pilocarpine model of epilepsy. Experimental Brain Research. 2013;**226**(2):153-163

[182] David Y, Cacheaux LP, Ivens S, Lapilover E, Heinemann U, Kaufer D, et al. Astrocytic dysfunction in epileptogenesis: Consequence of altered potassium and glutamate homeostasis? The Journal of Neuroscience. 2009;**29**(34):10588-10599

[183] Wong M, Ess KC, Uhlmann EJ, Jansen LA, Li W, Crino PB, et al. Impaired glial glutamate transport in a mouse tuberous sclerosis epilepsy model. Annals of Neurology. 2003;**54**(2):251-256

[184] Ueda Y, Doi T, Nagatomo K, Willmore LJ, Nakajima A. Functional role for redox in the epileptogenesis: Molecular regulation of glutamate in the hippocampus of FeCl3-induced limbic epilepsy model. Experimental Brain Research. 2007;**181**(4):571-577

[185] Lu Z, Zhang W, Zhang N, Jiang J, Luo Q, Qiu Y. The expression of glutamate transporters in chest compression-induced audiogenic epilepsy: A comparative study. Neurological Research. 2008;**30**(9):915-919

[186] Tessler S, Danbolt NC, Faull RL, Storm-Mathisen J, Emson PC. Expression of the glutamate transporters in human temporal lobe epilepsy. Neuroscience. 1999;**88**(4):1083-1091

[187] Akbar MT, Torp R, Danbolt NC, Levy LM, Meldrum BS, Ottersen OP. Expression of glial glutamate transporters GLT-1 and GLAST is unchanged in the hippocampus in fully kindled rats. Neuroscience. 1997;**78**(2):351-359

[188] Bough KJ, Paquet M, Pare JF, Hassel B, Smith Y, Hall RA, et al. Evidence against enhanced glutamate transport in the anticonvulsant mechanism of the ketogenic diet. Epilepsy Research. 2007;**74**(2-3):232-236

[189] Guo F, Sun F, Yu JL, Wang QH, Tu DY, Mao XY, et al. Abnormal expressions of glutamate transporters and metabotropic glutamate receptor 1 in the spontaneously epileptic rat hippocampus. Brain Research Bulletin. 2010;**81**(4-5):510-516

[190] Eid T, Lee TW, Patrylo P, Zaveri HP. Astrocytes and glutamine synthetase in epileptogenesis. Journal of Neuroscience Research. 2019;**97**(11):1345-1362

[191] Kong Q, Takahashi K, Schulte D, Stouffer N, Lin Y, Lin CL. Increased glial glutamate transporter EAAT2 expression reduces epileptogenic processes following pilocarpine-induced status epilepticus. Neurobiology of Disease. 2012;**47**(2):145-154

[192] Wetherington J, Serrano G, Dingledine R. Astrocytes in the epileptic brain. Neuron. 2008;**58**(2):168-178

[193] Swieboda P, Filip R, Prystupa A, Drozd M. Assessment of pain: Types, mechanism and treatment. Annals of Agricultural and Environmental Medicine. 2013;**Spec no. 1**:2-7

[194] Tao YX, Gu J, Stephens RL Jr. Role of spinal cord glutamate transporter during normal sensory transmission and pathological pain states. Molecular Pain. 2005;**1**:30

[195] Yang S, Chang MC. Chronic pain: Structural and functional changes in brain structures and associated negative affective states. International Journal of Molecular Sciences. 2019;**20**(13):3130

[196] Temmermand R, Barrett JE, Fontana ACK. Glutamatergic systems in neuropathic pain and emerging non-opioid therapies. Pharmacological Research. 2022;**185**:106492

[197] Ji RR, Nackley A, Huh Y, Terrando N, Maixner W.

Neuroinflammation and central sensitization in chronic and widespread pain. Anesthesiology. 2018;**129**(2):343-366

[198] Gegelashvili G, Bjerrum OJ. High-affinity glutamate transporters in chronic pain: An emerging therapeutic target. Journal of Neurochemistry. 2014;**131**(6):712-730

[199] Liaw WJ, Stephens RL Jr, Binns BC, Chu Y, Sepkuty JP, Johns RA, et al. Spinal glutamate uptake is critical for maintaining normal sensory transmission in rat spinal cord. Pain. 2005;**115**(1-2):60-70

[200] Wang W, Wang W, Wang Y, Huang J, Wu S, Li YQ. Temporal changes of astrocyte activation and glutamate transporter-1 expression in the spinal cord after spinal nerve ligation-induced neuropathic pain. The Anatomical Record (Hoboken). 2008;**291**(5):513-518

[201] Pereira V, Goudet C. Emerging trends in pain modulation by metabotropic glutamate receptors. Frontiers in Molecular Neuroscience. 2019;**11**:1-23

[202] Hewitt DJ. The use of NMDA-receptor antagonists in the treatment of chronic pain. The Clinical Journal of Pain. 2000;**16**(Suppl. 2):S73-S79

[203] Gegelashvili G, Bjerrum OJ. Glutamate transport system as a novel therapeutic target in chronic pain: Molecular mechanisms and pharmacology. Advances in Neurobiology. 2017;**16**:225-253

[204] Amin B, Avaznia M, Noorani R, Mehri S, Hosseinzadeh H. Upregulation of glutamate transporter 1 by clavulanic acid administration and attenuation of allodynia and hyperalgesia in neuropathic rats. Basic and Clinical Neuroscience. 2019;**10**(4):345-354

[205] Kristensen PJ, Gegelashvili G, Munro G, Heegaard AM, Bjerrum OJ. The beta-lactam clavulanic acid mediates glutamate transport-sensitive pain relief in a rat model of neuropathic pain. European Journal of Pain (London, England). 2018;**22**(2):282-294

[206] Eljaja L, Bjerrum OJ, Honoré PH, Abrahamsen B. Effects of the excitatory amino acid transporter subtype 2 (EAAT-2) inducer ceftriaxone on different pain modalities in rat. Scandinavian Journal of Pain. 2018;**2**(3):132-136

[207] Maeda S, Kawamoto A, Yatani Y, Shirakawa H, Nakagawa T, Kaneko S. Gene transfer of GLT-1, a glial glutamate transporter, into the spinal cord by recombinant adenovirus attenuates inflammatory and neuropathic pain in rats. Molecular Pain. 2008;**4**:65

[208] Yousuf MS, Kerr BJ. The role of regulatory transporters in neuropathic pain. Advances in Pharmacology (San Diego, Calif). 2016;**75**:245-271

[209] Hajhashemi V, Hosseinzadeh H, Amin B. Antiallodynia and antihyperalgesia effects of ceftriaxone in treatment of chronic neuropathic pain in rats. Acta Neuropsychiatrica. 2013;**25**(1):27-32

[210] Fontana IC, Souza DG, Souza DO, Gee A, Zimmer ER, Bongarzone S. A Medicinal chemistry perspective on excitatory amino acid transporter 2 dysfunction in neurodegenerative diseases. Journal of Medicinal Chemistry. 2023;**66**(4):2330-2346

[211] Limpert AS, Cosford ND. Translational enhancers of EAAT2: Therapeutic implications for neurodegenerative disease. The

Journal of Clinical Investigation. 2014;**124**(3):964-967

[212] Zhou Y, Danbolt NC. Glutamate as a neurotransmitter in the healthy brain. Journal of Neural Transmission (Vienna). 2014;**121**(8):799-817

[213] Kalivas PW. The glutamate homeostasis hypothesis of addiction. Nature Reviews. Neuroscience. 2009;**10**(8):561-572

[214] Christie MJ, Summers RJ, Stephenson JA, Cook CJ, Beart PM. Excitatory amino acid projections to the nucleus accumbens septi in the rat: A retrograde transport study utilizingd [3H] aspartate and [3H]GABA. Neuroscience. 1987;**22**(2):425-439

[215] Wise RA. Roles for nigrostriatal--not just mesocorticolimbic--dopamine in reward and addiction. Trends in Neurosciences. 2009;**32**(10):517-524

[216] Spencer S, Kalivas PW. Glutamate transport: A new bench to bedside mechanism for treating drug abuse. The International Journal of Neuropsychopharmacology. 2017;**20**(10):797-812

[217] Niedzielska-Andres E, Pomierny-Chamioło L, Andres M, Walczak M, Knackstedt LA, Filip M, et al. Cocaine use disorder: A look at metabotropic glutamate receptors and glutamate transporters. Pharmacology & Therapeutics. 2021;**221**:107797

[218] Griffin WC, Ramachandra VS, Knackstedt LA, Becker HC. Repeated cycles of chronic intermittent ethanol exposure increases basal glutamate in the nucleus accumbens of mice without affecting glutamate transport. Frontiers in Pharmacology. 2015;**6**:27

[219] Reissner KJ, Kalivas PW. Using glutamate homeostasis as a target for treating addictive disorders. Behavioural Pharmacology. 2010;**21**(5-6):514-522

[220] Sari Y, Smith KD, Ali PK, Rebec GV. Upregulation of GLT1 attenuates cue-induced reinstatement of cocaine-seeking behavior in rats. The Journal of Neuroscience. 2009;**29**(29):9239-9243

[221] Shen HW, Scofield MD, Boger H, Hensley M, Kalivas PW. Synaptic glutamate spillover due to impaired glutamate uptake mediates heroin relapse. The Journal of Neuroscience. 2014;**34**(16):5649-5657

[222] Abulseoud OA, Miller JD, Wu J, Choi DS, Holschneider DP. Ceftriaxone upregulates the glutamate transporter in medial prefrontal cortex and blocks reinstatement of methamphetamine seeking in a condition place preference paradigm. Brain Research. 2012;**1456**:14-21

[223] Sari Y, Toalston JE, Rao PS, Bell RL. Effects of ceftriaxone on ethanol, nicotine or sucrose intake by alcohol-preferring (P) rats and its association with GLT-1 expression. Neuroscience. 2016;**326**:117-125

[224] Niedzielska-Andres E, Mizera J, Sadakierska-Chudy A, Pomierny-Chamioło L, Filip M. Changes in the glutamate biomarker expression in rats vulnerable or resistant to the rewarding effects of cocaine and their reversal by ceftriaxone. Behavioural Brain Research. 2019;**370**:111945

[225] Sepulveda-Orengo MT, Healey KL, Kim R, Auriemma AC, Rojas J, Woronoff N, et al. Riluzole impairs cocaine reinstatement and restores adaptations in intrinsic excitability and GLT-1 expression. Neuropsychopharmacology. 2018;**43**(6):1212-1223

[226] Ciraulo DA, Sarid-Segal O, Knapp CM, Ciraulo AM, LoCastro J, Bloch DA, et al. Efficacy screening trials of paroxetine, pentoxifylline, riluzole, pramipexole and venlafaxine in cocaine dependence. Addiction. 2005; **100**(Suppl. 1):12-22

[227] Farahzadi MH, Moazen-Zadeh E, Razaghi E, Zarrindast MR, Bidaki R, Akhondzadeh S. Riluzole for treatment of men with methamphetamine dependence: A randomized, double-blind, placebo-controlled clinical trial. Journal of Psychopharmacology. 2019;**33**(3):305-315

[228] Itzhak Y, Martin JL. Effect of riluzole and gabapentin on cocaine- and methamphetamine-induced behavioral sensitization in mice. Psychopharmacology. 2000;**151**(2-3):226-233

[229] Tzschentke TM, Schmidt WJ. Blockade of morphine- and amphetamine-induced conditioned place preference in the rat by riluzole. Neuroscience Letters. 1998;**242**(2):114-116

[230] Besheer J, Lepoutre V, Hodge CW. Preclinical evaluation of riluzole: Assessments of ethanol self-administration and ethanol withdrawal symptoms. Alcoholism, Clinical and Experimental Research. 2009;**33**(8):1460-1468

[231] Kumar A, Singh A, Ekavali. A review on Alzheimer's disease pathophysiology and its management: An update. Pharmacological Reports: PR. 2015;**67**(2):195-203

[232] Sehar U, Rawat P, Reddy AP, Kopel J, Reddy PH. Amyloid beta in aging and Alzheimer's disease. International Journal of Molecular Sciences. 2022;**23**(21):12924

[233] de Paula VJR, Guimarães FM, Diniz BS, Forlenza OV. Neurobiological pathways to Alzheimer's disease: Amyloid-beta, TAU protein or both? Dementia & Neuropsychologia. 2009;**3**(3):188-194

[234] Hardy J, Cowburn R, Barton A, Reynolds G, Lofdahl E, O'Carroll AM, et al. Region-specific loss of glutamate innervation in Alzheimer's disease. Neuroscience Letters. 1987;**73**(1):77-80

[235] Mookherjee P, Green PS, Watson GS, Marques MA, Tanaka K, Meeker KD, et al. GLT-1 loss accelerates cognitive deficit onset in an Alzheimer's disease animal model. Journal of Alzheimer's Disease: JAD. 2011;**26**(3):447-455

[236] Woltjer RL, Duerson K, Fullmer JM, Mookherjee P, Ryan AM, Montine TJ, et al. Aberrant detergent-insoluble excitatory amino acid transporter 2 accumulates in Alzheimer disease. Journal of Neuropathology and Experimental Neurology. 2010;**69**(7):667-676

[237] Scimemi A, Meabon JS, Woltjer RL, Sullivan JM, Diamond JS, Cook DG. Amyloid-beta1-42 slows clearance of synaptically released glutamate by mislocalizing astrocytic GLT-1. The Journal of Neuroscience. 2013;**33**(12):5312-5318

[238] Meeker KD, Meabon JS, Cook DG. Partial loss of the glutamate transporter GLT-1 alters brain akt and insulin signaling in a mouse model of Alzheimer's disease. Journal of Alzheimer's Disease: JAD. 2015;**45**(2):509-520

[239] Kulijewicz-Nawrot M, Sykova E, Chvatal A, Verkhratsky A, Rodriguez JJ. Astrocytes and glutamate homoeostasis in Alzheimer's disease: A decrease

in glutamine synthetase, but not in glutamate transporter-1, in the prefrontal cortex. ASN Neuro. 2013;**5**(4):273-282

[240] Hogan DB. Long-term efficacy and toxicity of cholinesterase inhibitors in the treatment of Alzheimer disease. Canadian Journal of Psychiatry. 2014;**59**(12):618-623

[241] Zimmer ER, Kalinine E, Haas CB, Torrez VR, Souza DO, Muller AP, et al. Pretreatment with memantine prevents Alzheimer-like alterations induced by intrahippocampal okadaic acid administration in rats. Current Alzheimer Research. 2012;**9**(10):1182-1190

[242] Gettman L. Lecanemab-irmb (Leqembi™) for treatment of Alzheimer's disease. The Senior Care Pharmacist. 2024;**39**(2):75-77

[243] Zhu Y, Fotinos A, Mao LL, Atassi N, Zhou EW, Ahmad S, et al. Neuroprotective agents target molecular mechanisms of disease in ALS. Drug Discovery Today. 2015;**20**(1):65-75

[244] Trotti D, Aoki M, Pasinelli P, Berger UV, Danbolt NC, Brown RH Jr, et al. Amyotrophic lateral sclerosis-linked glutamate transporter mutant has impaired glutamate clearance capacity. The Journal of Biological Chemistry. 2001;**276**(1):576-582

[245] Barber SC, Mead RJ, Shaw PJ. Oxidative stress in ALS: A mechanism of neurodegeneration and a therapeutic target. Biochimica et Biophysica Acta (BBA) - Molecular Basis of Disease. 2006;**1762**(11):1051-1067

[246] Bruijn LI, Becher MW, Lee MK, Anderson KL, Jenkins NA, Copeland NG, et al. ALS-linked SOD1 mutant G85R mediates damage to astrocytes and promotes rapidly progressive disease with SOD1-containing inclusions. Neuron. 1997;**18**(2):327-338

[247] Van Den Bosch L, Van Damme P, Bogaert E, Robberecht W. The role of excitotoxicity in the pathogenesis of amyotrophic lateral sclerosis. Biochimica et Biophysica Acta. 2006;**1762**(11-12):1068-1082

[248] Cudkowicz ME, Titus S, Kearney M, Yu H, Sherman A, Schoenfeld D, et al. Safety and efficacy of ceftriaxone for amyotrophic lateral sclerosis: A multi-stage, randomised, double-blind, placebo-controlled trial. Lancet Neurology. 2014;**13**(11):1083-1091

[249] Li K, Hala TJ, Seetharam S, Poulsen DJ, Wright MC, Lepore AC. GLT1 overexpression in SOD1(G93A) mouse cervical spinal cord does not preserve diaphragm function or extend disease. Neurobiology of Disease. 2015;**78**:12-23

[250] Verche VL, Ikiz B, Jacquier A, Przedborski S, Re DB. Glutamate pathway implication in amyotrophic lateral sclerosis: What is the signal in the noise? Journal of Receptor, Ligand and Channel Research. 2011;**4**:1-22

[251] Walker FO. Huntington's disease. The Lancet. 2007;**369**(9557):218-228

[252] Massieu L, García O. The role of excitotoxicity and metabolic failure in the pathogenesis of neurological disorders. Neurobiology (Budapest, Hungary). 1998;**6**(1):99-108

[253] Arzberger T, Krampfl K, Leimgruber S, Weindl A. Changes of NMDA receptor subunit (NR1, NR2B) and glutamate transporter (GLT1) mRNA expression in Huntington's disease--an *in situ* hybridization study. Journal of Neuropathology and Experimental Neurology. 1997;**56**(4):440-454

[254] Estrada-Sanchez AM, Montiel T, Segovia J, Massieu L. Glutamate toxicity in the striatum of the R6/2 Huntington's disease transgenic mice is age-dependent and correlates with decreased levels of glutamate transporters. Neurobiology of Disease. 2009;**34**(1):78-86

[255] Todd AC, Hardingham GE. The regulation of astrocytic glutamate transporters in health and neurodegenerative diseases. International Journal of Molecular Sciences. 2020;**21**(24):9607

[256] Frank S. Treatment of Huntington's disease. Neurotherapeutics. 2014;**11**(1):153-160

[257] Assous M, Had-Aissouni L, Gubellini P, Melon C, Nafia I, Salin P, et al. Progressive parkinsonism by acute dysfunction of excitatory amino acid transporters in the rat substantia nigra. Neurobiology of Disease. 2014;**65**:69-81

[258] Chotibut T, Davis RW, Arnold JC, Frenchek Z, Gurwara S, Bondada V, et al. Ceftriaxone increases glutamate uptake and reduces striatal tyrosine hydroxylase loss in 6-OHDA Parkinson's model. Molecular Neurobiology. 2014;**49**(3):1282-1292

[259] Yadav A, Collman RG. CNS inflammation and macrophage/microglial biology associated with HIV-1 infection. Journal of Neuroimmune Pharmacology. 2009;**4**(4):430-447

[260] Afaf E-A, Hussain AD. Biomarkers-Directed Strategies to Treat Autism. In: Mu W, Frank AW, editors. Role of Biomarkers in Medicine. Rijeka: IntechOpen; 2016. p. Ch. 10

[261] Takahashi KK. Glutamate transporter EAAT2: Regulation, function, and potential as a therapeutic target for neurological and psychiatric disease. Cellular and Molecular Life Sciences: CMLS. 2015;**72**(18):3489-3506

[262] Chen JX, Yao LH, Xu BB, Qian K, Wang HL, Liu ZC, et al. Glutamate transporter 1-mediated antidepressant-like effect in a rat model of chronic unpredictable stress. Journal of Huazhong University of Science and Technology Medical sciences = Hua zhong ke ji da xue xue bao Yi xue Ying De wen ban = Huazhong keji daxue xuebao Yixue Yingdewen ban. 2014;**34**(6):838-844

[263] Nakagawa T, Kaneko S. SLC1 glutamate transporters and diseases: Psychiatric diseases and pathological pain. Current Molecular Pharmacology. 2013;**6**(2):66-73

[264] Sorensen MF, Heimisdottir SB, Sorensen MD, Mellegaard CS, Wohlleben H, Kristensen BW, et al. High expression of cystine-glutamate antiporter xCT (SLC7A11) is an independent biomarker for epileptic seizures at diagnosis in glioma. Journal of Neuro-Oncology. 2018;**138**(1):49-53

[265] Huberfeld G, Vecht CJ. Seizures and gliomas - towards a single therapeutic approach. Nature Reviews. Neurology. 2016;**12**(4):204-216

[266] Werner P, Pitt D, Raine CS. Multiple sclerosis: Altered glutamate homeostasis in lesions correlates with oligodendrocyte and axonal damage. Annals of Neurology. 2001;**50**(2):169-180

[267] Parkin GM, Udawela M, Gibbons A, Dean B. Glutamate transporters, EAAT1 and EAAT2, are potentially important in the pathophysiology and treatment of schizophrenia and affective disorders. World Journal of Psychiatry. 2018;**8**(2):51-63

[268] Escobar AP, Wendland JR, Chávez AE, Moya PR. The neuronal

glutamate transporter EAAT3 in obsessive-compulsive disorder. Frontiers in Pharmacology. 2019;**10**:1362

[269] Takahashi K, Foster JB, Lin CL. Glutamate transporter EAAT2: Regulation, function, and potential as a therapeutic target for neurological and psychiatric disease. Cellular and Molecular Life Sciences. 2015;**72**(18):3489-3506

Chapter 5

The Role of Glutamate in Pathogenesis of Brain Edema in Intracerebral Hemorrhage

Vladimir Rendevski and Boris Aleksovski

Abstract

This chapter is dedicated to the impressing molecule of glutamamte—both an amino acid and a major excitatory neurotransmitter in the brain. The chapter focuses scientific on review of our work in the past decade, stressing the role of glutamate excitotoxicity as significant and sensitive biomarker for quantification of the volume of brain edema in intracerebral hemorrhage, which is important in the trajectory of clinical deterioration. We explain several developed mathematical models based on multiple regression analysis for the purposes of prognostication and potential clinical implications. These mathematical models can contribute to clinical decision making and resolving the dilemma between conservative and operative treatment in patients with hemorrhagic stroke, especially in the first 4–5 days.

Keywords: glutamate, prognostication, brain edema, intracerebral hemorrhage, excitotoxicity, clinical implications

1. Introduction

Almost all living organisms on the planet use glutamic acid in protein biosynthesis. This incredible molecule is an α-amino acid and is a non-essential nutrient for humans due to the ability of our body to synthesize enormous quantities of glutamic acid needed for building protein blocks—the main building blocks of our cells. The molecular formula of glutamic acid is C_5H_9NO (symbol Glu or E), and its systematic IUPAC name is 2-aminopentanedioic acid. Nevertheless, glutamic acid is more known for its anionic form—glutamate ($^{-}OOC - CH(NH_3^{+}) - (CH_2)_2 - COO^{-}$), which naturally occurs in the body under physiological pH values.

Glutamate is the major constituent of a wide variety of proteins and is considered as one of the most abundant amino acids in the human body [1]. Nevertheless, besides its involvement in protein synthesis, glutamate plays a crucial role as the main "master" excitatory neurotransmitter in both the central and peripheral nervous systems [2]. Glutamatergic transmission is the major excitatory transmission, accounting for over 90% of the synaptic connections in the human brain, and its pathways highly interconnect with numerous other neurotransmitter pathways [3]. Glutamate is produced within the central nervous system through the conversion of glutamine in the glutamate-glutamine cycle, facilitated by the enzyme glutaminase [4]. This conversion takes place either within the presynaptic neuron or in nearby glial cells. Glutamate receptors are also distributed extensively broadly across neurons and glial cells throughout the brain and spinal cord. Moreover, glutamate also serves as the precursor for the synthesis of gamma-aminobutyric acid (GABA), the chief inhibitory neurotransmitter in the brain, catalyzed by the enzyme L-glutamic acid decarboxylase [5] in the GABAergic neurons.

Glutamate influences biological processes by attaching to and stimulating receptors on the post-synaptic cell surface. Mammals possess four categorized families of these receptors [6]: amino-3-hydroxy-5-methyl-4-isoxazolepropionic acid AMPA receptors (GluA1–GluA4), kainate receptors (GluK1–GluK5), N-methyl-D-aspartate NMDA receptors (GluN1, GluN2A–GluN2D, GluN3A, and GluN3B), and metabotropic glutamate receptors. The first three families are ionotropic glutamate receptors (ligand-gated ion channels), that is, integral membrane proteins composed of four large subunits that form a central ion channel pore [6]; glutamate binding activates these channels by opening them, enabling ion passage, and thus stimulating fast excitatory neurotransmission. In contrast, the metabotropic family consists of G protein-coupled receptors (mGluR), which exert their effects through second messengers such as diacylglycerol and cAMP [1].

Given its dual role as an amino acid and neurotransmitter, glutamate serves a diverse range of vital physiological functions. Studies strongly suggest that glutamate is critical for sustaining optimal energy levels essential for numerous CNS functions, especially neuroplasticity, which is vital for adapting to environmental changes [2]. Consequently, disruptions in glutamate function can have significant repercussions in both disease and injury contexts.

2. The role of glutamate in pathological conditions: a focus on intracerebral hemorrhage (ICH)

Many studies point out also to the crucial roles of glutamate in several pathological conditions. The harmful effect of glutamate on the CNS was first observed in 1954 by Dr. Takashi Hayashi (Keio University School of Medicine, Tokyo), a Japanese scientist who detected the occurrence of motor deprivation as a result of the direct effect of glutamate on the CNS. This report went unnoticed for several years until 1957, when the toxicity of glutamate was highlighted again by D. R. Lucas and J. P. Newhouse. They proved this by applying a subcutaneous injection of monosodium glutamate in newborn mice, and subsequently determined the destruction of neurons in the inner layers of the retina [7].

Later, in 1969, John Olney discovered that the damage was not limited to the retina, but also to other parts of the CNS, and he introduced the term excitotoxicity. He also postulated that cell death is limited to postsynaptic neurons that have receptors for activation by glutamate agonists and that damage can be prevented by blocking these agonists [8].

Excitotoxicity is a pathological process through which nerve cells are damaged and destroyed due to excessive stimulation by foreign neurotransmitters, such as glutamate and similar substances. Pathophysiologically, excessive activation of glutamate receptors in the CNS (NMDA and AMPA receptors) occurs as a result of increased glutamate levels, and consequently activation of the mechanism of excessive uptake of calcium ions (Ca^{2+}) in the cell [9]. The latter, in turn, activates several intracellular enzymes, such as phospholipase (PLC), endonuclease, protease, which secondarily damages the cellular structure (components of the cytoskeleton, cellular membrane, and DNA).

Many studies stress the role of glutamate as an excitatory neurotransmitter in the pathogenesis of cerebral ischemia [10]. Confirmation for this association are many experimental studies in which glutamate antagonist drugs were applied, where a reduction in the volume of the infarcted region occurs. The usefulness of the glutamate antagonist is based on the hypothesis that excitotoxicity persists at least for several hours after the occurrence of a stroke [11].

Increased levels of glutamate and consequent excitotoxic effect on the CNS, except in ischemic cerebrovascular insults, have also been detected in other pathological conditions, such as traumatic brain and spinal cord injuries, hearing loss due to exposure to excessive noise or ototoxicity, and neurodegenerative diseases of CNS (multiple sclerosis, Alzheimer's disease, amyotrophic lateral sclerosis (ALS), and Huntington's and Parkinson's disease) [12, 13]. Other conditions that were shown to cause increased levels of CNS glutamate are alcoholism, hypoglycemia, and status epilepticus [14, 15].

It is particularly important to emphasize that, unlike cerebral ischemia and traumatic brain injury where glutamate-induced excitotoxicity role in triggering cell death, its contribution to the development of brain injury was well documented, and its role in intracerebral hemorrhage (ICH) was not clearly defined in patients before 2015 [16]. The first findings of elevated extracellular glutamate levels after ICH were obtained using *in vivo* brain microdialysis techniques in experimental animals with induced ICH. Namely, a fourfold increase in glutamate was detected ipsilateral to the hematoma at 30 min after ICH, and these levels also remained elevated for 5 h [17]. Similarly, only a few studies have examined the role of blocking glutamate accumulation on brain damage after ICH. Mendelow [18] suggested that the NMDA receptor antagonist D-CPP reduces edema in rats. Also, in animal models of ICH with collagenase, it was shown that the non-competitive antagonist of NMDA receptors —memantine, causes a decrease in hematoma expansion, a decrease in cell death, and a decrease in infiltration of immune cells [19]. These results indicate that excitotoxicity may be an important mechanism for cell death after ICH. Later, Sharp et al. [20], using a genomic approach, identified a 20-fold increase in the expression of a member of the Src family—Lyn in the brain after ICH, which deals with the regulation of NMDA receptors through phosphorylation. Based on this, they suggested that ICH induces thrombin production after hemorrhage, which results in Src activation, which contributes to NMDA receptor phosphorylation, leading to neuronal damage. Nevertheless, although some authors suggested that certain mechanisms through which glutamate contributes to ICH-induced brain damage were specific [21], and differed from those in ischemic damage, and there were no data in human patients with ICH. It seemed that glutamate-triggered excitotoxicity contributes to secondary brain damage in ICH, but the interaction with the other mechanisms of brain damage, especially inflammatory processes, was not well investigated.

There is considerable evidence to support the theory of TNF-α involvement in the development of perifocal edema. In the brain, TNF-α is synthesized by microglia and astrocytes, while TNF-α receptors are found on glial cells and neurons. Although TNF-α has neuromodulatory abilities in the healthy brain, its function in the post-ICH brain is clearly neurotoxic and detrimental [22]. One of the factors leading to an increase in the brain level of TNF-α after ICH is the production of thrombin during hematoma formation [23, 24], and thrombin directly stimulates the production of TNF-α. Elevation of TNF-α levels causes activation of microglial cells and astrocytes after the injury, regulation of blood-brain barrier permeability, glutaminergic transmission, and synaptic plasticity [22]. After brain injury in experimental animals, elevated levels of TNF-α were detected in the tissue adjacent to the injury site, which contributes to the development of edema through the increased permeability of the blood-brain barrier. In addition, TNF-α increases excitatory synaptic transmission *via* elevated AMPA receptor expression and reduces inhibitory transmission, thus causing excitotoxicity [25]. In summary, there is rational preclinical evidence that increased TNF-α concentrations have detrimental effects on the brain after ICH, involving glutamate excitotoxicity. Based on the proposed model, TNF-α causes additional release of glutamate from synaptosomes, as well as inhibition of glutamate reuptake from the synaptic cleft back to the presynaptic neuron, causing excitotoxicity. Therefore, there is a possibility of an interaction effect between excitotoxicity and inflammatory mechanisms in the development of brain secondary injury, but before 2018, there were no studies examining this interaction effect (whether it is additive, synergistic, antagonistic, etc.).

Studies on peripheral glutamate levels in patients with ICH are very rare. In this context, for example, Castillo et al. showed significant differences in glutamate levels between patients with good and poor neurological outcomes [26], but this study did not include a control group for comparison of their values.

Tanphaichitr et al. [27] reported reference values of peripheral glutamate levels of 22.4 ± 3.2 nmol/mL glutamate in the blood plasma of healthy individuals, while according to Tsai and Huang [28], the values were estimated as 33.2 ± 15, 4 μmol/L. In the same study, the authors point out that the concentration of blood plasma glutamate is one of the lowest compared to other amino acids, but also one of the most constant, that is, with the least degree of variability in terms of the diet [28].

The study by Rendevski et al. [29] of our research group aimed to evaluate the role of peripheral plasma glutamate and TNF-α levels as biomarkers for ICH. Furthermore, to examine the prognostic role and possible interactions of these variables in the development of edema volume 5 days after ICH. The study was based on the hypothesis that since an increased variability of the blood-brain barrier (BBB) is a typical result after ICH [30], the excitotoxic and pro-inflammatory mediators can transfer from the brain in the blood and be detected peripherally. In this study, significantly higher blood plasma glutamate and TNF-a levels were detected in ICH patients at admission, when compared to healthy controls, which stresses the importance of these mediators in the pathology of the ICH. The glutamate values were more than threefold increase in patients (median value of 107.75 μmol/L) when compared to the median of the healthy population analyzed in the study (31.13 μmol/L)—a value very similar to those reported by Tsai and Huang [28]. Since the difference in glutamate levels between healthy individuals and patients with ICH was striking, it was concluded that glutamate is an important molecular marker of excitotoxicity, the concentration of which increases significantly immediately after the onset of intracerebral hemorrhage. In North Macedonia, no study results of reference values of glutamate in human plasma have been published so far; namely, these were also the first results for reference values for glutamate in the healthy human population.

The study also showed that the anatomic localization of ICH (lobar/deep; left/right hemisphere) did not influence the influx of glutamate and TNF-α and equally induced excitotoxicity and inflammation, regardless of ICH position. Glutamate levels within the patient group did not differ significantly between males and females, or between the different age groups. Moreover, it was demonstrated that the symptom severity and the initial volume of ICH were the major drivers for the variability of the glutamate levels in patients with ICH.

Peripheral glutamate levels were shown as significant predictors for the formation of brain perifocal edema 5 days after ICH [29]. Namely, it was demonstrated that glutamate and TNF-α independently contribute (without any effect of interaction) to the development of the edema, regardless of the localization of the ICH. This was a very important discovery since the worst deterioration in ICH patients occurs due to the formation of brain perifocal edema, a well-proven factor of mortality and poor outcomes after ICH. Hence, aiming at the prevention of formation of large edema volumes in patients after ICH, the ability to predict its formation is crucial benefit.

The later study by Rendevski et al. [31] has also separated glutamate as an independent and significant predictor of development of the brain perifocal edema. This study focused on advanced 3D modeling for prediction and quantification of the perihematomal brain edema formation after ICH. Several 3D models and interactive plots were constructed, which could accurately predict 77% of the variability in the volumes of the edema within patients of ICH. The model was focused on glutamate and TNF-α, suggesting the primary role of excitotoxic and inflammatory mechanisms in the secondary brain damage and the pathogenesis of the edema. The model was also characterized by very high significance (one-way ANOVA resume: $F = 33.7592$, $^{*}p = 7.4 \cdot 10^{-19}$), and with good overall characteristics and fit.

The proposed equation for mathematical quantification of the edema was given as:

$$V_{\text{edema}} = 0.3292 \cdot c_{TNF-\alpha} + 0.2484 \cdot c_{\text{glutamate}} + 0.3162 \cdot V_{ICH} + 1.6299 \cdot CSS + 0.9283 \cdot c_{\text{glucose}} - 49.4949 + a \quad (1)$$

where *a*—summarizes the effects of anatomic localization and the presence of diabetes (**Figure 1**).

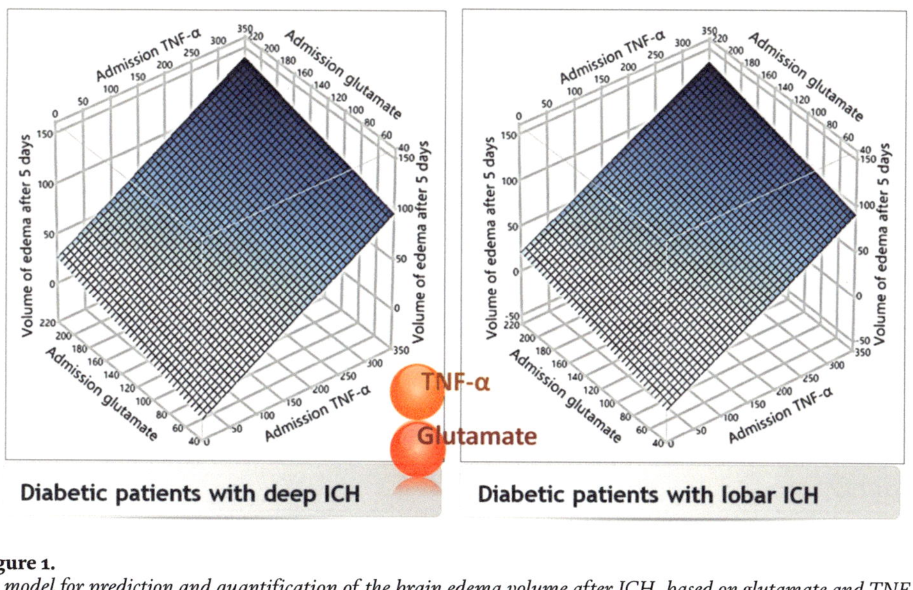

Figure 1.
3D model for prediction and quantification of the brain edema volume after ICH, based on glutamate and TNF-α values. The model summarizes the differences in prognostication between deep and lobar ICH, within ICH diabetic patients.

3. Conclusions

The necessity for urgent care of patients presenting in the emergency department with intracerebral hemorrhage is undeniable. The worst neurological deterioration in these parents was associated with the formation of perifocal brain edema, a proven predictor for poor outcome, and peripheral glutamate levels resulting from excitotoxicity-induced ICH were shown as a promising marker for edema prediction. The constructed glutamate-based models and the developed interactive plots for prediction of the formation of the brain edema could be beneficial for clinical decision-making between conservative treatment and surgical intervention, especially in the group of threatened ICH patients where high volumes of the edema are expected to occur during the parent's hospitalization trajectory. In summary, since glutamate-mediated excitotoxicity was one of the proven mechanisms operating during ICH, monitoring of the peripheral glutamate plasma levels, originating from the brain *via* the disrupted blood-brain barrier, can tell a lot about the severity of the insult and its possible progression, mainly in the "evolution" of edema development.

Author details

Vladimir Rendevski[1]* and Boris Aleksovski[2]

1 Medical Faculty, "Ss. Cyril and Methodius" University, University Clinic of Neurosurgery, Skopje, North Macedonia

2 Faculty of Natural Sciences and Mathematics, "Ss. Cyril and Methodius" University, Skopje, North Macedonia

*Address all correspondence to: vladimirrendevski@yahoo.com

References

[1] Meldrum BS. "Glutamate as a neurotransmitter in the brain: Review of physiology and pathology" (PDF). The Journal of Nutrition. 2000;**130**(4S Suppl):1007S-1015S. DOI: 10.1093/jn/130.4.1007s

[2] Pal MM. Glutamate: The master neurotransmitter and its implications in chronic stress and mood disorders. Frontiers in Human Neuroscience. 2021;**15**:722323. DOI: 10.3389/fnhum.2021.722323

[3] Niciu MJ, Kelmendi B, Sanacora G. Overview of glutamatergic neurotransmission in the nervous system. Pharmacology, Biochemistry, and Behavior. 2012;**100**(4):656-664. DOI: 10.1016/j.pbb.2011.08.008

[4] Zhang D, Hua Z, Li Z. The role of glutamate and glutamine metabolism and related transporters in nerve cells. CNS Neuroscience & Therapeutics. 2024;**30**(2):e14617. DOI: 10.1111/cns.14617

[5] Le Vo TD, Kim TW, Hong SH. Effects of glutamate decarboxylase and gamma-aminobutyric acid (GABA) transporter on the bioconversion of GABA in engineered Escherichia coli. Bioprocess and Biosystems Engineering. 2012;**35**(4):645-650. DOI: 10.1007/s00449-011-0634-8

[6] Traynelis SF, Wollmuth LP, McBain CJ, Menniti FS, Vance KM, Ogden KK, et al. Glutamate receptor ion channels: Structure, regulation, and function. Pharmacological Reviews. 2010;**62**(3):405-496. DOI: 10.1124/pr.109.002451

[7] Lucas DR, Newhouse JP. The toxic effect of sodium L-glutamate on the inner layers of the retina. A.M.A. Archives of Ophthalmology. 1957;**58**(2):193-201

[8] Olney JW. Brain lesions, obesity, and other disturbances in mice treated with monosodium glutamate. Science. 1969;**164**(3880):719-721. DOI: 10.1126/science.164.3880.719

[9] Manev H, Favaron M, Guidotti A, Costa E. Delayed increase of Ca^{2+} influx elicited by glutamate: Role in neuronal death. Molecular Pharmacology. 1989;**36**:106-112

[10] Rothman SM, Olney JW. Glutamate and the pathophysiology of hypoxic–ischemic brain damage. Annals of Neurology. 1986;**19**:105-111. DOI: 10.1002/ana.410190202

[11] Muir KW, Lees KR. Clinical experience with excitatory amino acid antagonist drugs. Stroke. 1995;**26**:503-513

[12] Kim AH, Kerchner GA, Choi DW. In: Marcoux FW, Choi DW, editors. Section I Mechanic Approaches to CNS Neuroprotection. New York: Springer; 2002. pp. 3-36

[13] Hughes JR. Alcohol withdrawal seizures. Epilepsy & Behavior. 2009;**15**:92-97. DOI: 10.1016/j.yebeh.2009.02.037

[14] Camacho A, Massieu L. Role of glutamate transporters in the clearance and release of glutamate during ischemia and its relation to neuronal death. Archives of Medical Research. 2006;**37**:11-18. DOI: 10.1016/j.arcmed.2005.05.014

[15] Fujikawa DG. Prolonged seizures and cellular injury: Understanding

the connection. Epilepsy & Behavior. 2005;7:3-11. DOI: 10.1016/j.yebeh.2005.08.003

[16] MacLellan C, Peeling J, Colbourne F. Cytoprotection strategies for experimental intracerebral hemorrhage. In: Carhuapoma R, Mayer SA, Hanley DF, editors. Intracerebral Hemorrhage. Cambridge: Cambridge Univ Press; 2010. pp. 217-227

[17] Qureshi AI, Ali Z, Suri MFK, et al. Extracellular glutamate and other amino acids in experimental intracerebral hemorrhage: An in vivo microdialysis study. Critical Care Medicine. 2003;**31**:1482-1489. DOI: 10.1097/01.CCM.0000063047.63862.99

[18] Mendelow AD. Mechanisms of ischemic brain damage with intracerebral hemorrhage. Stroke. 1993;**24**:115-119

[19] Lee S-T, Chu K, Jung K-H, et al. Memantine reduces hematoma expansion in experimental intracerebral hemorrhage, resulting in functional improvement. Journal of Cerebral Blood Flow and Metabolism. 2006;**26**:536-544. DOI: 10.1038/sj.jcbfm.9600213

[20] Sharp F, Liu DZ, Zhan XAB. Intracerebral hemorrhage injury mechanisms: Glutamate neurotoxicity, thrombin, and Src. Acta Neurochirurgica. 2008;**105**:43-45

[21] Keep RF, Hua Y, Xi G. Intracerebral haemorrhage: Mechanisms of injury and therapeutic targets. Lancet Neurology. 2012;**11**:720-731. DOI: 10.1016/S1474-4422(12)70104-7

[22] Mccoy MK, Tansey MG. TNF signaling inhibition in the CNS: Implications for normal brain function and neurodegenerative disease. Journal of Neuroinflammation. 2008;**5**:45. DOI: 10.1186/1742-2094-5-45

[23] Lee KR, Kawai N, Kim S, et al. Mechanisms of edema formation after intracerebral hemorrhage: Effects of thrombin on cerebral blood flow, blood-brain barrier permeability, and cell survival in a rat model. Journal of Neurosurgery. 1997;**86**:272-278. DOI: 10.3171/jns.1997.86.2.0272

[24] Hua Y, Wu J, Keep RF, et al. Tumor necrosis factor-alpha increases in the brain after intracerebral hemorrhage and thrombin stimulation. Neurosurgery. 2006;**58**:542-550; discussion 542-50. DOI: 10.1227/01.NEU.0000197333.55473.AD

[25] Behrouz R. Re-exploring tumor necrosis factor alpha as a target for therapy in intracerebral hemorrhage. Translational Stroke Research. 2016;**7**:93-96. DOI: 10.1007/s12975-016-0446-x

[26] Castillo J, Davalos A, Alvarez-Sabin J, et al. Molecular signatures of brain injury after intracerebral hemorrhage. Neurology. 2002;**58**:624-629. DOI: 10.1212/WNL.58.4.624

[27] Tanphaichitr V, Leelahagul P, Suwan K. Plasma amino acid patterns and visceral protein status in users and nonusers of monosodium glutamate. The Journal of Nutrition. 2000;**130**:1005S-1006S

[28] Tsai PJ, Huang PC. Circadian variations in plasma and erythrocyte concentrations of glutamate, glutamine, and alanine in men on a diet without and with added monosodium glutamate. Metabolism. 1999;**48**:1455-1460

[29] Rendevski V, Aleksovski B, Stojanov D, Aleksovski V, Rendevska AM, Kolevska M, et al. Peripheral glutamate and TNF-α levels in patients with intracerebral hemorrhage: Their prognostic values and interactions toward the formation of the edemal

volume. Neurologia i Neurochirurgia Polska. 2018;**52**(2):207-214. DOI: 10.1016/j.pjnns.2017.10.003. Epub 2017 Oct 19

[30] Rost NS, Greenberg SM, Rosand J. The genetic architecture of intracerebral hemorrhage. Stroke. 2008;**39**:2166-2173. DOI: 10.1161/STROKEAHA.107.501650

[31] Rendevski V, Aleksovski B, Mihajlovska RA. Advanced 3D modelling for prediction and quantification of the perihematomal brain edema formation after intracerebral haemorrhage: Implications of biochemical, radiological and clinical variables. In: 59th International Neuropsychiatric Congress, Mind & Brain, Pula, Croatia. Zagreb, Croatia: International Institute for Brain Health; 2019. p. 145